Your Health is Your Choice

Health Made Simple

Dennis Richard

ISBN: 1468021737
ISBN-13: 9781468021738
Library of Congress Control Number: 2011962156
CreateSpace, North Charleston, SC

Contents

Additional Pictures and videos that may be of interest are posted on my websites, www.DRhealthclub.com and www.YourHealthisYourChoice.org. They are referenced as they relate to each chapter.

Foreword

My reason for writing this book is to explain just how simple and inexpensive health can be.
Health Made Simple

Anyone with an open mind and reads the true stories of how I reversed my many health issues and my aging process over the past 20 years will realize it is within all our power to do the same. This book offers hope for all to see how I have made health simple and affordable for nearly everyone.

I say *nearly* everyone, because I often recall one of Henry Ford's more famous quotes: "There are those that think they can do something, and there are those that think they can't do it, and they are both right." The limiting factor is our mind: our belief in our own ability to learn what we need to know to make our health our choice!

This book can potentially help everyone to understand that health can be very simple when we learn a few things that will allow the immune system to function at its optimum potential. Only the body can heal itself; we just need to give it a chance. Drugs are not the answer to achieving this goal. There is no drug on the market today without a downside: more drugs will be needed to counteract its harmful effects.

Accepting that only the body can heal itself was the start of my incredible path to resolving my many health issues. This fact has allowed me to go from feeling 90 years old and that my life was over to feeling better than I did when I was in my twenties. In 1991, I was diagnosed with prostate cancer; in addition, I had many other health issues, including a ruptured disk in my neck that prevented me from working most of my last year and a half on the fire department. I felt that I was dying, and I was in so much pain that I just didn't care.

Once I learned that the underlying cause of nearly all health issues is some form of pathogen or environmental toxin, I did a thorough cleansing and detoxing, followed by the right nutrition and a little exercise. My body did heal itself from every disease and health issue I had when I retired from the fire department in 1991.

The information I have learned from dozens of doctors I have spoken with and/or whose lectures I have listened to at health trade shows has worked for me. Health really can be just that simple.

I feel that God has blessed me with this knowledge and the ability to make this my reality, and it is my obligation to share my accomplishments with all who are guided to read it.

Acknowledgments

For all of those who have directly or indirectly helped me with my book through what they taught while guiding me through the successful reversal of many health issues, I want to express my sincere gratitude. They helped me compile the documentation of my health issues.

To Bonnie Morgan: I might never have finished this book without the help and encouragement of a very special lady with her extraordinary organizational ability. She arranged approximately 3,000 pages of my notes from the past 20 years, which were scattered over hundreds of documents and computer files, and categorized the information into chapters. She then encouraged me to go through them and write my book.

To Jo Cipra: I might never have started without her help. She was there to guide me on the first steps to regain my health through cleansing and detoxing. She was determined to research and tell me about all the different cleanses and making sure I followed the directions to the letter. I might not even be here today if she hadn't given me confidence in my ability to learn what I needed to know to change my life.

A special thanks to Nikki Benjamin and Dr. Sal D'Onofrio for all of their help in rewriting this book and correcting my many mistakes. They have both been very helpful in so many ways. I just can't thank them enough.

I am very grateful to one of the smartest people I know, Geoff Norrena, who has been very diligent in checking my facts and correcting things I was not stating in the most understandable way. While at health shows, I often get excited when I hear a doctor make a statement that is hard to believe. I explain to Geoff what I think I heard, and he often will say politely, "What you think you heard may not be what the doctor thought he said!" We both get a laugh out of that while Geoff explains to me what the doctor wrote on his website. A lot of what I know is through Geoff's research, since he is so diligent in checking the facts and making sure that I understand what I thought I had learned.

I want to thank my youngest son, Don Richard, for his design of my book cover. Many times he has been very helpful with his great ideas and his graphic design ability. He has always been there for me anytime I have needed his assistance. His promotional ideas along with his artistic abilities have been a great help to me ever since he graduated from college nearly 20 years ago. I am very fortunate to have a large, loving family that has all been very supportive through all of my health issues.

To Linda Hathaway, one of my closest friends, I owe a great deal of gratitude for helping me in so many ways in reversing some of my more serious health challenges. She has taught me so much about health and has given me a spiritual awareness that has made a big difference in my life.

Among the many people who have made the biggest difference in my life, contributed a great deal to my knowledge, and helped me in reversing my many health issues are Ed S., Ed H. Jim Humble, Dr. Dean Bonlie, Dr. Howard Hagglund, Dr. Sal D'Onofrio, Dr. Stephen and Beth Daniel of Quantum Techniques, Dr. William Hitt, Dr. John Humiston, Dr. Hulda Clark, Dr. Richard S., Dr. Deborah Banker, Dr. Bradley Nelson, Dr. Tom Hesselink, Dr. Donald Brown, Dr. Wade Sol, Dr. Jesse Partridge, Bob Beck, and Dr. Tony O'Donnell. They have all become friends and have been very kind with their time and with their patience in teaching me much of what I know. I also want to mention one of my closest friends, Jay Lashlee; what he has taught me has enabled me to understand what I have learned from the above-listed friends. A few people wish not to be named for personal reasons, and I believe it is because of fear of the Food and Drug Administration (FDA).

What Dr. Bonlie has taught me about magnetic therapy has really changed and improved my life. He likely saved my life, or at the least, gave me back a life worth living. My chapter on magnets is not to be missed. The healing power of magnets is incredible. I now understand the meaning of Dr. Becker's book, *Body Electric*, and have some idea about how and why subtle energy can help (and harm) the body.

This book is about the things I have tried and how they worked or did not work for me. I have complete faith that I will find answers to any future health issues, as I have been successfully guided to overcome all I have had so far.

CHAPTER 1

My Story

My story is about going from feeling 90 years old with many health problems to feeling 20 with few health issues. Now health seems simple, as does anything we understand. My expectation is that by the time you finish my book, health will seem as simple to you as it does to me. I truly believe that *Your Health is Your Choice*.

In 2005, Dr. William Hitt, MD, a psychiatrist and PhD in microbiology, explained to me that weight control is simple once we understand that nearly every overweight person has a fungal issue. Fungi have a unique ability to manipulate our brain chemistry, making us crave the food they want to eat. I met Dr. Hitt when I was quite overweight. I craved chocolate, ice cream, and many other high-fat, high-sugar foods. Within 4 days of following his protocol, I had lost all craving for these foods, and within 6 months, I had lost about 60 pounds without counting calories or depriving myself of anything. Once I lost my cravings, I found that my body gravitated to a normal, healthy weight naturally without dieting. I do think that my improved diet had a lot to do with it as well, since I changed from eating 80 percent meat to about 80 percent salads, fruits, and vegetables during that time. When the body is receiving a balanced nutritional diet, it helps reduce cravings as well; we no longer have the desire to eat more and more as our body attempts to meet its nutritional needs.

Addictions, whether to tobacco, alcohol, food or something else, are most often caused by fungus. When we address the physical problem of fungal overgrowth, the cravings are gone and the remaining emotional aspect of addiction can then be successfully addressed through AA, Al-Anon, and psychotherapy. Dr. Stephen Daniel and Dr. Bradley Nelson both work with the emotional releases very successfully once the physical cravings are gone.

When I retired in 1991, I weighed 310 pounds. When I met Dr. Hitt in 2005, I was down to 270 pounds. It was a 15 year struggle just to lose 40 pounds. After following Drs. Hitt and Humiston's candida protocol, I lost the next 60 pounds in 6 months with little effort. Dr. Hitt and Dr. Humiston were right on. Without cravings for the first time in 45 years, I had enough willpower to achieve my desired weight.

I have been able to maintain this weight now for the past 5 years with little effort. I have not had any cravings now that I understand how to eat and prevent any further fungal issues.

Shortly after joining the fire department in 1961, I read in a fire department trade magazine that the life expectancy for a fireman was 58 and that the average firefighter lived only 2 years after retirement. This short life span was primarily due to smoke and toxic chemical exposure that damaged the hearts and lungs of many firefighters.

I officially retired August 1, 1991, but had been unable to work the last year and a half before my retirement. I was in such pain that I felt as if I was dying, and I didn't care. It seemed I had so many health issues, including senility (fungus can be a major contributor to this as well), which made it difficult to think clearly enough to search for possible solutions to any of my health issues. I was certain at that time that if a doctor couldn't fix me, nothing could be done; health seemed beyond my comprehension. I started on my journey around the world seeking the best health information I could find. I was driven to unlock the secrets of health; I was certain my life depended on it.

I had wanted to be a fireman from the time I was very young. In 1956, while still in high school, I volunteered at the age of 15.

At that time, firemen were only paid around $350 a month and worked 72 hours a week. In spite of that, I loved the feeling of satisfaction when helping others in need. After 3 years in the U.S. Marine Corps (USMC), I was employed at the fire department in 1961. We were only paid $402 a month and still worked 72 hours a week. We were so poorly educated that most of us smoked cigarettes to "build up a tolerance to smoke." Being an ex-Marine and determined to "eat more smoke" than anyone I worked with, I smoked 4 packs of unfiltered Camels a day for several years. By the time I was 28 years old, I found myself hyperventilating just walking up one flight of stairs, which forced me to quit smoking for good. My stamina subsequently improved. Though a limited number of air packs were available to firemen in the early years, the importance and value of them to our health and safety were not realized until the catastrophic MGM Grand fire in 1980, where 87 people died.

About a year and a half before completing my 30 years of service, I ruptured a disk in my neck while fighting a large fire. It left me in constant pain for several years. More than a dozen medical doctors and therapists told me there was nothing they could do for me. I was given only a 10 percent chance of improvement and a 70 percent chance I'd be in worse shape if they operated on me. They told me that I would have to learn to live with the pain.

I had also developed a hiatal hernia. For several years, I slept sitting up because I had extremely severe heartburn when I lay in a flat position. No matter how many antacids I took, such as Mylanta, Tums, or Rolaids, they did not help. I went for several years without a good night's sleep, which I believe had a devastating effect on my overall health.

In addition, I had developed chronic prostatitis over the preceding 10 years. Several urologists prescribed antibiotics for 3–6 months at a time. The last one kept me on this medication for a full year and then said, "Tough luck—it will eventually become cancerous." It already had, yet this doctor didn't pick it up. Another did, just a few months later. I was told I would most likely live only 2–5 years.

These three problems culminated about the same time. I felt that my life was over. I was in constant pain from my neck injury along with symptoms of fibromyalgia; I gained 40 pounds; and I wanted to do nothing but eat, sleep, and watch TV. At that time, I hurt so much I didn't care whether I lived or died. I had seen over 20 different doctors by this time, many of whom were specialists in different fields, and they all told me the same thing: "Accept it, learn to live with the pain, it is a part of getting old; and if you're lucky, you'll get to live another 10 or 15 years." I thought: in this pain, I just don't want to live any longer at all.

I was sick and tired of being sick and tired, and the medical doctors offered no hope at all. I felt I was dying, and it seemed the doctors were doing more to kill me than to cure me with all the medication I was given. I had to make a choice: would I give up on life or would I pursue all means to health? I chose health and began my road to recovery.

Through prayer, God has continually brought people into my life who have guided me every step of the way. With every health issue I have faced, someone has come into my life and taught me things I could do for myself. I have been able to reverse one health issue after another, thus finally realizing that **my health really is my choice.**

This book contains information about what we can do for ourselves that will allow us optimum health. I feel certain that we can all successfully treat ourselves for any and all diseases. Hundreds of people I have talked to have successfully treated themselves as I have done for many of the same conditions, along with many more than I have experienced. The only difference between me and most others is that I documented most of my conditions and wrote about what I have overcome, along with what worked and did not work for me.

There are many great doctors, scientists, and researchers who are discovering new supplements and technology, such as energy healing, which work far better than standard medical procedures. Some of these methods seem to have benefits that exceed all possible limits. Nevertheless, the American Medical Association

(AMA), and the U.S. Food and Drug Administration (FDA), prohibit medical doctors from utilizing many of them. Our only opportunity to access most of these complementary and alternative methods and modalities is to do it ourselves. Once I realized that only my body could heal itself, it just needed a little help through cleansing and detoxing. By getting the environmental toxins out of my body and reducing my body's viral and fungal load along with the other pathogens, I began feeling much better. Then when I added a little exercise and gave my body the right nutrients to allow my immune system to do its job, the results were phenomenal and health became simple to me.

I have researched many forms of alternative and complementary health care for my own personal benefit. Once I started on my road to recovery and realized I didn't have to be sick and tired or live in constant pain, I became obsessed with learning more and more about health. Having spent much more money than I could afford on different products and health care devices, I realized that some worked, but many didn't. Yet I felt years younger than I did at the time of my retirement. I realized that my improvement was directly related to my increase in knowledge. The more health trade shows I attended, and the more doctors and health care professionals I had the opportunity to speak to about my health issues, the better I got.

I now feel certain I will live to be at least 150 years old, and I believe I will never have another sick day in my life. I believe this is within everyone's reach. That was my belief in June of 2009, but more important than how long I live is the quality of life that I will enjoy. Good health does not have to cost a lot of money. Once we give our immune system what it needs to heal and work at its maximum potential, we all can know the peace of mind I now experience.

Health starts in the mind! Negative thoughts cause undue stress on the subconscious mind, which stresses the whole body and its immune system. To be truly happy and maintain peace and harmony, our mind, body, and soul must be in balance.

Back in the 1950s, fire department high school volunteers were paid 25 cents an hour, and we received 2 high school elective credits for on-the-job training as well if we lasted a year. We would work from 5:00 p.m. to 7:00 a.m. every other night and 24 hours at a time on the weekends and holidays. This was a win-win situation for the City of Henderson, Nevada, and the young guys as well. It gave us the opportunity to learn many things about life that few of us had access to prior to this experience.

Education: It is not always what we learn but how we learn it that allows us to use it for our benefit and the benefit of others. This experience made a very big impact on my life, and I owe a great deal of gratitude to many men I worked with in my tough early years. Unfortunately, I didn't realize how they helped shaped my life at the time, and I often didn't express my gratitude as I wish I had. I would like to thank them all for their time and effort in making me the person I am today. Working as a volunteer fireman along with my tour of duty in the USMC taught me far more about life than school did. I was 30 years old before I realized how important a rounded education was, and I was greatly lacking in that. I started college while I worked at the fire department, receiving Associate in Arts Degrees (AA) in fire science and business management.

Shortly after retiring, I started following Dr. Hulda Clark's protocols for cleansing and detoxing as described in her book, *A Cure for All Cancer.* When I started with the colon cleanse in 1993, I lost 30 pounds just by eliminating disease-causing build-up in my colon. However, I also thought she was extreme at the time. She went so far as to recommend we get rid of carpeting in the home, and I had just put in new carpet throughout. I was not about to take it all out, but as time went on and I continued to get very good results from her cleanses, I finally did get rid of most of my carpet.

We don't destroy our health overnight, and we don't get it back overnight either. I heard a well-known lecturer at a health trade show state that for every 7 years we neglect our health with poor diet and lifestyle, it takes one year of doing everything right to reverse it.

I believe that is most likely true; however, in my case, I had abused myself for 30 years by eating and drinking anything I wanted with no regard to any detrimental effects it might have. It then took 16 years to learn and to improve my circumstance by doing a little here and there, plus 4 additional years, to go from feeling 90 to 20 years old.

In 1993, I started with Dr. Hulda Clark's colon cleanse, and I lost thirty pounds just by eliminating the disease-causing buildup in my colon. It removed the bad parasites (e.g., *Candida albicans*) which were eating holes through my intestine. The parasites, which everyone has, are normally held in check by our friendly flora. You see, only 6 percent to 7 percent of the pathogenic bacteria in our body are harmful, and many of them have a beneficial purpose when held in check. But when a doctor puts us on antibiotics, it kills everything indiscriminately. The harmful pathogens are stronger, so the few that are left come back fast, as they are no longer outnumbered (nearly twenty to one) by the friendly flora.

If the harmful pathogens are not stopped in time, they will eat many holes in your intestine (a "leaky gut syndrome"). Your body then becomes overwhelmed with toxins leaking into your lymph fluid and blood, and you become sick and tired. Many doctors still treat symptoms; when I wrote this in 1993 as part of my notes, they were still trained to prescribe more antibiotics when people came down with a fever. More antibiotics will just add fuel to the fire. They will temporarily stop the bacterial infection but not a yeast or viral infection. You will feel better for a while; but each time you repeat the scenario, you will get worse from overuse of antibiotics. I am pleased to say that today, most doctors are more aware of the problem and most are no longer abusing antibiotics as they did at the time this was written nearly 20 years ago.

In the year 2011, as I look back on the past 20 years of my life, I have come to realize that I have accomplished what few others have, in regard to health. It is not that I am all that smart; I believe it is because I have been divinely guided in my pursuit. I feel that this is my purpose: to share what I have received in learning how to restore and rebuild my own health.

It seems as though every prayer, in which I have asked for something to help me in this effort, has been answered. I feel I have manifested not only my own health improvements, but the opportunity to do something to give my life meaning and purpose—a purpose that would benefit humanity and allow me to help make the world a better place to live.

I also realized that nearly every day (in addition to thanking God for my wonderful family), my prayers included my wish to raise my children to be more knowledgeable and better prepared for a healthy life than I was. I always felt I could help change the world by teaching them to have a good work ethic, to always stand by their word, and to be honest in thought and deed. I wanted them to always be kind and helpful to everyone that comes into their lives, to live in love and forgiveness to all, and enjoy a successful, happy life.

My grandmother taught me when I was quite young that "as long as people are breathing, they have problems, and most people feel theirs are more important and overwhelming than others'." She went on to say: "Walk a mile in someone else's shoes and never judge anyone, as God will judge you as you judge others." I have remembered her words hundreds of times throughout my life, and it became important for me to pass on that knowledge to my children. To me, this meant appreciating life's lessons no matter how painful they may seem at the time. By doing what is in the best interest of all, for the highest and best good for all concerned, we will always do the right thing. For whatever reason, we may need to endure certain experiences; appreciating their lessons will help us grow into the exceptional people we wish to become. I can't help but be proud that all of my children have exceeded my hopes and expectations.

I am so proud of all of my children and am delighted that each one of them married someone who fits perfectly into the family and are all each other's best friends. Thankfully, all of my prayers have been answered in the past, and I have no doubt that this will continue for the rest of my life.

In 1960, realizing the power that computers have to allow us to compound our knowledge, I felt certain my life expectancy would be at least 150 years. My expectation was that our government and the medical schools would use this for the benefit of all. Now I realize, if not for the personal computer and the Internet, my vision would never have come to pass. Money and corruption may prevent millions of people from having the opportunity to learn what has allowed me to make my health my choice. We can never allow the government to control the Internet and suppress knowledge, which would keep us in the dark about how simple health truly is.

In 2010, I feel 20 years old and am now looking forward to the next 100-plus years. Not only have I been able to regain my health and vitality, my weight and waist measurements are the same as when I was 20. Never having had the willpower to diet and exercise, I understand how energy works and realize that my prayers, positive thinking, and not allowing negative thoughts and energy to enter my mind have enabled me to successfully manifest what I have become today.

I thrive on job satisfaction and accomplishment, but it is interesting to note that my past jobs have provided very little of them for me. I would get a tremendous feeling of satisfaction from helping save someone's life or property with the fire department, but that only occurred 2 or 3 times a year. Most of the time, the opportunity to be of service for those in need was not there for me, since there were so many other firemen at the scene of most emergencies. What I did as an individual was of little consequence, so it was seldom that I received that feeling of job satisfaction. What I do today by sharing the stories of my success in reversing my many health issues is far more rewarding than anything I have done in my past. Nearly every day, one or more people call me, thanking me for helping them with their health issues.

Working with 28% sodium chlorite solution, also known as Miracle Mineral Supplement (MMS), has opened many doors and brought many exceptional people into my life. These people have been kind enough to share their knowledge and stories of success with me. By educating and allowing me to continue to learn, they provided me with information that I can share for the benefit of many others. My life has become so exciting, filled with not only endless opportunity but a spiritual evolution that has been helped by the use of Sodium Chlorite (MMS). It has given me clarity of thought that I haven't experienced since I was a young man. I believe this is the primary reason I am 100 percent pain free now, after living in pain for most of my life.

Many doctors state that the primary cause of bodily pain is the lack of oxygen at the cellular level and the cells' inability to excrete their waste. This causes inflammation, which in turn causes pain, and this combination reduces blood flow leading to an internal environment creating a breeding ground for pathogens. Sodium Chlorite (MMS) seems to address both of these issues, so I believe it is the main reason I am now pain free.

I have used Jim Humble's protocol for taking Sodium Chlorite (MMS) for 5 years now. I brush and floss my teeth with it, and my bleeding gums stopped within 4 days. I have not had my teeth cleaned in nearly 6 years now, and I have absolutely no plaque on my teeth. This is because Sodium Chlorite (MMS) has oxidized the plaque from my teeth. When your gums are healthy, it is much easier to stay in overall good health.

My main purpose, and most important point in writing this book, is to let you know that answers exist today that allow all of us to successfully treat ourselves for any and all sicknesses and diseases. We can learn to reduce or eliminate most pain. It doesn't matter what our problem is; we can accomplish this through our own education. This is another reason I feel compelled to write: to give everyone hope and the understanding that most health issues are simple and inexpensive for us to treat ourselves.

The United States has, by far, the world's most expensive medical treatments, yet we do not rank in the top 20 of the world's healthiest nations. Now we can use the Internet to access information on new and old medical treatments, so we can take our health into our own hands. Methods such as Rife, ozone, and magnetic therapy are overlooked by "conventional" medicine. Not everything on the Internet is credible, so I would like to help guide you through the maze of information and undo the brainwashing we've received during the course of our lives by some people in the American medical community and big pharmaceutical companies.

In June 2011, I had the opportunity to meet and listen to Dr. Matthias Rath, MD, lecture at a health trade show in Las Vegas, Nevada. He explained that most heart disease and cancer has been curable for 20–30 years, and it has been suppressed. He has been publishing his research for more than 20 years now, doing his best to bring this information to light. He is world renowned and has the support of nearly everyone who has taken the time to evaluate his research. His research proves this is possible because proper nutrition works, and he points out the harmful effects of pharmaceutical drugs. You would think our government would want to make this information available to everyone, as it has the potential to fix our broken health care system and reduce our national debt.

He went on to explain he has been sued 110 times by different government agencies and big pharmaceutical companies around the world. If I understood correctly, he has never lost a case, because his scientific research is undeniable. I have known about Dr. Rath for over 5 years now, and I have used some of his products, as I still have some minor heart issues remaining, according to my doctor. He brought me to tears as he spoke of his desire to make a difference in the world. He did not complain about his trials and tribulations; he just stated the facts about what has happened to him and many others.

After his lecture, there were many people wanting to speak to him. I waited in line for the opportunity to meet him and shake his hand to thank him for his service to humanity. I found myself continually wiping the tears from my eyes at the thought of the sacrifices he has made for all of us. He is obviously a brilliant man, and far above most of us with his research, knowledge, and determination to do the right thing: fighting the pharmaceutical industry to bring this information to light. We spoke for about 15 minutes as if we were the only two people in the room, and I found him very humble in his manner and speech. He emanated a spiritual energy that I had only experienced a few times before in my life.

He has a plan that can change the world, and I want to be a part of it. I hope everyone in the world will want to be a part of it as well. I plan to do all I can to support his efforts to bring his work to everyone's attention. His plan is simple, as it needs to be to bring people together.

Dr. Matthias Rath's plan is to provide educational material to every health food store around the world, making them educational centers that explain just how simple health can be. Through cleansing, detoxing, and nutrition, our body can and will heal itself of nearly all diseases.

My website will have a link to his information. You can find both sites by going to: www.YourHealthisYourChoice.org or www.DRhealthclub.com

Live in love and light, and be the change you wish to see in the world.

CHAPTER 2

Chelation Therapy–the first step in reversing my health issues and my aging process

Chelation was the start of my recovery process. At the time of my retirement from the fire department in 1991, I was so feebleminded I could not have a conversation without forgetting my point. I would ask 20–30 times a day, "What was I saying? What were we talking about?" I couldn't complete a prayer without forgetting what I wanted to thank God for. My mother and grandmother were both diagnosed with Alzheimer's disease at that time, and I was as bad off as they were.

Quite often in my conversations with my grandmother, I was the one telling her how old age really sucks; and she was nearly 50 years older than I. She would laugh at the thought, but I was serious! I suffered from short-term memory loss and senility, which added to my belief that my life was about over. I believe my brain fog was largely due to my exposure to toxic chemicals and metals over 30 years on the fire department. My eyesight was getting worse, and I had been wearing bifocals for 20 years. In addition, I had tinnitus, a constant ringing in my ears that often drove me crazy.

I first heard about chelation therapy in 1987 during a trip to Micronesia. I was fascinated with the idea of getting my mind back so I could better enjoy what I believed to be the last couple of years of my life. I had always been attracted to the South Pacific islands. I really wanted to see them before I died.

On the first full day of my trip, I met Pamela de Maigret and her sister Tammy Painter. It turned out that we all had tickets on the Continental Airlines "island hopper" for the same dates and times. We flew from island to island and became good friends, sharing the cost of taxis, car rentals, and boats.

I noticed something different about Pamela and her ability to recall. Her memory amazed me. Every profession has its own terminology that allows its members to share information better, but it didn't matter whether we were talking to a nuclear scientist, a geologist, or a botanist; no matter how well educated they were or whether they had no education at all, she unconsciously related to that person effortlessly in her conversation. She rarely had to think about any subject; she just joined in the conversation like an old friend talking about something familiar. Her vocabulary was beyond that of any person I had ever met and has remained so, 20 years later.

After a few days of observing her in these different conversations, I asked her, "Is it your IQ that allows you to fit into these situations, or are you taking some sort of supplements that give you seemingly total recall?" She appeared to be completely unaware of her unique ability. 2 or 3 days went by. We discussed the subject again, and she told me about taking chelation therapy. She said, "It is an intravenous (IV) solution that takes about 3 hours per treatment. It is supposed to clean the circulatory system and remove the toxins and heavy metals from the brain." She went on to say that the benefits were so subtle that she hadn't really noticed any significant change at the time, but after thinking about it, she did feel her memory had improved.

I wrote down the term "chelation" since I had never heard of it before and wanted to learn more about it. After returning from my trip, I forgot all about it and had lost my notes. Pamela sent me a letter and some information about chelation and the names of two doctors in Las Vegas who did the therapy. I was really surprised that she remembered to do this, as more than a month had passed since the trip.

I called both doctors and my insurance company to find out the cost and see if the insurance would pay any part of it. It would not. Since I couldn't afford $120 per treatment then, and not knowing for sure whether it would have benefited me, I put it off.

Everywhere I travel, I ask everyone I meet which country he or she enjoyed most. Where would he or she most like to go back? A lot of people told me about Costa Rica, so I decided to take a short trip there to check it out. Fortunately, I have a daughter who worked for an airline, which made air travel affordable for me.

I was very fortunate to have checked into a bed and breakfast called Lisa-Tec. It is on a beautiful golf course close to San Jose, the capital of Costa Rica, and is owned by an American woman named Lisa. It just so happened that the next morning, she was going for a chelation treatment. It was half the price as in the States, and after listening to Lisa describe how it had benefited her, I had to go along.

Doctor Solano fit me right in with Lisa and several others. It was nice to go where you can talk and share experiences with others; it makes the 3-hour treatment go by fast. One of the guys I met at that first appointment was 80 years old. He told me that 4 weeks earlier, he could hardly walk the 50 or 60 feet from the car into the doctor's office, and he could not drive himself, either. He had previously had a couple of angioplasties (balloon procedures) and triple-bypass heart surgery. By his 7th chelation treatment, in less than a month he was walking 2–3 miles a day and was able to drive on his own.

I ended up staying 2 weeks and undergoing 6 treatments. It was really "crossing the line" by talking Dr. Solano into doing 3 treatments a week. 2 a week should be the maximum, but I was going back to the States soon and my body was handling them well. On my last treatment, I could feel a pain in my kidneys and wished I had taken my doctor's advice. I would not recommend that anyone take more than 2 chelation treatments per week, because they put a real strain on the kidneys and deplete a lot of the body's minerals.

I have since used the following information to achieve similar results. It is much less expensive and more convenient, as it can be done at home. In addition, there is the added potential benefit of getting many micronutrients scientists have not even discovered yet that I believe are present.

I found that most companies and health food stores sell powdered rock source minerals, many of which the body cannot assimilate. The body can only utilize a small portion of these minerals. They add more stress on the kidneys, since they have to eliminate so much of them as waste. Actually, all minerals are inorganic by nature, but plants are able to make them organic through their digestion. Now in an organic form, the body readily accepts them as food.

I am so thankful that I found a source of minerals that duplicate nature and are created by organic media. At angstrom size, they are 99.99 percent bioavailable at the cellular level in liquid form. These minerals do not need to be chelated to fool the body into accepting them, or have to be broken down to get their benefits. In the right form and at the right size, they are ionic and seen by our bodies as organic. These are Trace Minerals, distributed by www.A2ZHealthProducts.com. Until I found them, I thought all minerals came from rocks. I now realize that we can get virtually all of our minerals from this source and these are far more beneficial for our health.

Humic and fulvic acid are two other sources of liquid minerals that are not well known but that have many incredible health benefits that few people realize at this time. they are found in ancient sinkholes containing vegetation from centuries ago that have not been exposed to our toxic environment. The fulvic acid liquid molecule is extremely small. The body loves it; it is able to break down heavy metals in the cells. Humic acid is a big-brother molecule that can lock on to the heavy metals and pull them out of our cells without letting go. These two can be lifesaving for many people.

I believe that I was able to pull out heavy metals, chemicals, and radiation by taking these forms of minerals and that I rebalanced my body in a very short time. I like to take the Humic and Fulvic acids during the day in distilled water without chlorine, and then I take the Trace Minerals at night, without dilution.

I have spoken to many people who use HUMIC X-1 to chelate heavy metals out of the body. This product only pulls heavy proton metals and does not pull out needed body-friendly minerals. I have had people tell me they got their lives back after a short time using this form of mineral.

I received 4 very unmistakable benefits from my first 6 chelation treatments. There was a noticeable improvement in my eyesight, and the tinnitus was gone. My energy level went up a lot, and most important of all, I quit saying that old age really sucks—because my short-term memory had improved a great deal.

Extremely excited about my improvements, I came home and sold an investment property for a lot less than it was worth just to get the cash to allow me to return to Costa Rica. On my first visit back to Dr. Solano's office, I met my 80-year-old friend once again, and he was on his 30th treatment. He told me he was feeling so good that he had just ordered $3,000,000 of new gold mining equipment and planned to go back to work.

Deeply inspired by his story, along with stories from several other patients who all had great success, I was determined to stay as long as it would take to reverse my health problems. This time I stayed for 3 months and took a total of 30 treatments. By the end of the 3 months, I had a tremendous improvement in my memory and my whole thought process.

My energy level was back up, and I started walking a lot. I remember one special day during the rainy season: I was wearing a brand new pair of shoes, and I must have walked 5 or 6 miles in the rain when my shoes completely fell apart. I really liked those shoes; they were the most expensive ones I had ever bought. It just felt so good walking in the warm rain. Even without an umbrella or raincoat, I just didn't want to stop walking.

My eyes continued to improve as well. I only needed to wear my glasses in poor light or if the print was really fine. I didn't need to use them at all for driving or flying, and my sight seemed to be back to 20/20.

The tinnitus was gone on my first trip after the 6 treatments, but when I got home and started back on my high-fat, high-sugar diet, it came back within a few days. It is hard for me to believe now, but I didn't associate it with my diet at that time. After my second trip and my second round of treatments, I noticed that the ringing was gone. In addition to taking the chelation treatments, I had the tendency to eat more like a Costa Rican—a lot of fresh fruits, vegetables, chicken, and fish, along with black beans and rice. I learned to enjoy that diet while there, but I didn't seem to stick with it at home.

I have found that I can control my tinnitus through diet alone. Since I have type O blood, I must eat meat, according to the book, *Eat Right for Your Blood Type,* by Dr. Peter J. D'Adamo. I have tried a lot of different diets and have found that without sufficient meat and protein in my diet, I won't last more than a few days before I start to feel weak and often shaky. If you have a problem with weight or just want to improve your diet, I recommend you read this book. It will help you understand your body's nutritional needs as it relates to your specific blood type.

There are many other ways of losing weight and helping your body to chelate naturally, if we have the time and willpower. A proper diet can do wonders, and I have since found an oral chelation formula that I use for maintenance. When we wait until there is a major health problem before taking action, as most of us do, we often have to take drastic steps to get beyond the emergency. I have been using humic acid for chelation; several doctors and health care professionals have recommended it to me. It seems to be working very well to maintain an ongoing cleanse and rid my body of the contamination we are exposed to daily.

I feel very fortunate that things worked out well for me. This was my first step in accepting responsibility for my own health. Doors started opening that allowed me to understand, accept, and treat my own health problems successfully. I found it was to my advantage not to have much understanding of health, because

I didn't have a lot of preconceived ideas of what should and shouldn't work. I have since remained open-minded to everyone's thoughts and suggestions. Since I have tried many things with little expectation of any benefit, often I find myself surprised to see an improvement with whatever issue I was trying to address.

Once I saw the incredible benefits of chelation for myself, I was so eager to learn and understand more and was open to everyone's ideas of what I might try. When you're open to listening and learning, it is amazing the people you attract into your life that are willing to help and share their knowledge. By the time I started studying universal law, I had already experienced the law of attraction; that opened my eyes to my ability to attract some of the world's top health care professionals, who have shared their knowledge with me. The saying "When the pupil is ready, the teacher will appear!" is exactly what happened to me.

After my 30 sessions of IV chelation, I had my mind back and could think once again. After many other health improvements, I ended up hosting *Health Talk Radio* on KLAV in Las Vegas 5 days a week, 1 hour a day, for 2 years. I interviewed nearly everyone who had written a book on alternative health. Wayne Dyer was one of the most memorable I interviewed; he made me realize that I had not set out to have a radio show that gave me access to so many incredible people. It's true: I didn't plan it but unconsciously manifested it because of my desire to learn all I could about health. This interview led me to a whole new understanding of my reason for living, my purpose in life. It is to help the world to become a better place for all. That has been my prayer for the past 20 years now; I am living my dream as I share what I have learned. My expectation is that I will give people hope, because no matter what they're told about their health condition, it is just another person's opinion. It is your own opinion that counts, and only you can make a difference in your life, since only your body can heal itself. That is why *Your Health is Your Choice.*

Even though I could think clearly, felt better, could see better, and the ringing in my ears was gone, I was still sick and tired a great deal of the time and in pain from the ruptured disk in my neck. I was also diagnosed with prostate cancer. That really got my attention, but my attitude had changed with my previous successes. Now I was looking for answers so I could take my next step on the road to recovery.

Understanding chelation: It may help you to understand chelation as a form of cleansing. It cleanses your circulatory system, which includes your arteries, veins, and capillaries. It removes plaque and heavy metals, and your whole body receives the benefit. This was my first experience at cleansing, and the benefit was so remarkable that I started looking at what else I could do to cleanse my body.

I could write a book on all the cleansing I have done, as I have gone from one cleanse to another for nearly 20 years now. We have 10 organs (or organ systems); they all need cleansing, and not just one for each. We shower every day—well, most people do, as they understand the need to keep the outside of their bodies clean—but we need to understand that our inside is even more important to keep clean. With our increasingly toxic environment, it is more important now than ever.

I tried several different types of oral chelation and several herbal products that were reported to have chelating properties, with no noticeable benefits from either. This isn't to say that none of them work; it's just that I didn't seem to get any perceptible benefit. It's possible that had I taken higher doses or stayed on them longer, they may have worked.

In 1997, I met Dr. Dan Royal, DO (a doctor of osteopathic medicine) in Henderson, Nevada, where his practice is located. I told him of my experience with chelation, and he told me he uses it with his patients with a great deal of success. He highly recommended I try more treatments.

I received about 10 more treatments and felt my health was back to where it had been after my first 30 treatments in Costa Rica 5 years earlier. Dr. Royal took a lot more scientific approach to his treatment plan; he had blood, urine, and several other tests done before he started the series of treatments.

I do love Costa Rica, and I highly recommend people visit there. I also recommend a stay with my friend Lisa Carney, as she has a beautiful place on the Cariari golf course and the price is less than half of the cost of a hotel. It is an easy walk to the hotel for a meal or the casino. In addition to being a great hostess, Lisa is the best resource for anything you may want to buy, if you want to rent a car, or have any other needs, and she is among the funniest people I know. I have a notebook filled with Lisa's words of wisdom that has kept me entertained for many hours over the past years, as I have stayed with her on nearly every trip I have made to Costa Rica; she can be reached at lisatec1@hotmail.com.

In 2002, I had 3 heart attacks caused by blockages; I was able to clear them with the use of a combination of IV chelation, dimercaptosuccinic acid (DMSA), other oral chelation methods, and ozone. This combination worked very well for me; within 3 months, an angiogram showed my blockages were all gone.

During the first part of February 2007, I had once again noticed a decline in my short-term memory as well as my eyesight; it had been several years since my last series of chelation treatments. Fortunately, I met Jim Humble in Mexico, and he explained the benefits of Sodium Chlorite (MMS). Once I understood that it was an *oxidizing agent*, it made sense to me how it would help cleanse my circulatory system. Within a few weeks, I noticed a tremendous improvement in my eyesight, my short-term memory, and energy level, just as I had previously experienced using chelation.

It blew my mind to find out that I got the same benefit from my first $20 bottle of Sodium Chlorite (MMS) as I had from the thousands of dollars I had previously spent on IV chelation. I got many other health benefits as well. In other chapters I will cover how and why it works.

I am not suggesting that you don't need chelation at all, because Sodium Chlorite (MMS) does not chelate; it oxidizes, so you get a similar benefit from a different approach. It is my opinion, however, that chelation has benefits that the oxidation process may not be able to duplicate.

It is very easy to become depressed and give up on life when you can't think and you have no idea of where to start to turn your health around. My goal is to give hope to all who are guided to read my story, as I can't imagine a health issue I won't be able to reverse. Even if I died tomorrow from an accident or a health issue, my journey has been worth the hardships and heartaches; my quality of life has been incredible for the past few years.

I love feeling 20 years old once again. Health truly is simple. My health is my choice, and *Your Health is Your Choice.* Only you can make a difference in your life, and it starts with your education and the understanding that only your body can heal itself, we just need to give it a chance.

CHAPTER 3

Ozone Therapy and Other Oxidative Therapies

Ozone and magnetic therapy are the two most important therapies I have studied and used to restore my health. The unifying cause of all disease is disturbance of function, an imbalance in the internal environment. Once anyone understands that the underlying cause of most disease is some form of pathogen or environmental toxin that disturbs cellular function, health becomes simple. Oxidative therapies can address both, even if the health issue is not directly related. Removing the pathogens and toxins helps our body heal itself. The use of oxidation allows our immune system to be more effective and efficient in healing whatever the problem may be.

Oxygen is essential to all human, animal, and plant life; in fact, to nearly all life on earth. It is a vital nutrient for all healthy, living cells. The use of ozone appears to go beyond the benefits of oxygen in the treatment of disease. There are few books written on this subject in the United States, so it is difficult to learn the many ways ozone can be used in restoring our health.

The best known book on the subject that I have read and that was written and published in the United States is *O_2xygen Therapies* by Ed McCabe. I highly recommend this book to anyone who wants to better understand the benefits of ozone as a therapy.

Mother Nature cleanses and purifies the air with ozone. That fresh, clean, invigorating scent that you often smell after a summer thunderstorm is ozone. The chemical symbol for oxygen is $O_{2;}$ the large O stands for oxygen, and the small $_2$ means that the oxygen molecules are gathered together in clusters of 2. In ozone, the molecules of oxygen are grouped together in clusters of 3 (or more) and are represented by the symbol O_3.

Health Benefits of Ozone

- Ozone has been proven to kill viruses in donated blood samples.
- Cancer researchers report ozone intolerance in tumor cells.
- Many viruses are vulnerable to ozone, including herpes, Epstein-Barr, influenza, mumps, measles, and HIV.
- Ozone oxidizes fibrous tissue in veins and hemorrhoids, allowing them to shrink to their normal size, recede into the tissue, and improve circulation. Varicose veins and hemorrhoids may disappear.
- Ozone treatments revitalize and rejuvenate people who are healthy, thus helping prevent the onset of disease.
- *The above information was taken from my notes collected in different lectures over the years, and I do not have a specific source. I do believe it is all true from my personal experiences.*

Most ozone treatments are given to otherwise healthy people to revitalize and rejuvenate their health and prevent disease. However, ozone is a powerful sanitizer. It kills nearly every known pathogen, including common bacteria, viruses, molds, and fungi. Ozone is also one of the most effective deodorizers known. In contrast to chlorine, ozone actually improves the taste and odor of water. The FDA has approved ozone for use in sanitizing foods and surfaces that contact foods. In fact, ozone is approved for use on foods that are labeled as "organic." This means that an "organic" apple can be washed with ozonized water and remain an "organic" apple. When used as directed, the high concentration of ozone in water will kill 99.9 percent of E. coli, salmonella, or other pathogens on the surface of the food. Ozone not only kills germs on food, it has also been shown to extend shelf life. Washing foods in ozonized water kills decay-causing bacteria on the surface. In addition, ozone destroys ethylene gas, which acts as a ripening agent in fruits and vegetables.

Is ozone safe? It has proven highly effective in the treatment and elimination of more than 40 common diseases with no toxic side effects. Doctors that understand how to safely use ozone, characterize it as nontoxic and harmless. There are strict guidelines for protocols involving safe levels for both short and long term exposure. In many applications, ozone is dissolved in water to make it safe to use and easy to handle. There are no defined exposure limits for ozone in water, as it is generally regarded as safe.

Note: Dr. Humiston's statement after reviewing this chapter regarding the paragraph on ozonating apples:

Yes, ozone will kill everything at high doses, but you cannot use those high doses in your body without killing your cells , also. So don't give the impression that ozone IV can kill 99% of microbes, because it doesn't. That's what you have to change in your writing.

Also, it would be good for you to include a paragraph about the different ways of administering ozone, to make things clear: IV, in water for drinking, body bag.

Over the last 20 years, I have listened to and taken numerous notes from many doctors and health care professionals who spoke about the use of ozone and its effects on the human body. I believe that all I have written to be true based on my personal use of ozone, and the benefits I have experienced. I have heard different doctors state that there are more than 50 ways to use ozone to improve our health. I could spend a month or two going through my notes looking for examples, and writing many pages on this subject alone. Hopefully, Dr. Humiston's comments above will encourage you to search for yourself to find options that will work best for you.

More information about my personal use of ozone is discussed in my heart and liver chapters and in others chapters as well. I also explain the way Dr. Hitt and Dr. Humiston used it in Tijuana, Mexico, for many years. There are many ways to use ozone that will benefit our immune system; in my opinion, these two exceptional medical doctors are among the best in the world.

In 1992, I was skeptical at first about ozone therapy; because it seemed too good to be true, but I decided to buy an ozone machine with a bag and try it myself. No clothes are worn in an ozone bag, because they collect the ozone and prevent it from being absorbed through your skin. The more exposed skin in the bag, the faster oxygen can enter your blood. Your head must be kept out of the bag and away from any leakage of ozone from the bag, because we cannot breathe concentrated ozone. It will "burn" our lungs.

When ozone is introduced into the bag in high concentrations, the O_3 molecules break down into O_2 and O_1. The O_2 molecules are electron balanced, meaning that they are not free radicals. The O_1 is a positively charged nucleus looking for electrons. The O_1 is very energetic and in correct circumstances, can pass through the skin. Upon entering the bloodstream, they can pair up with other O_1 molecules to form O_2. The O_1 molecule can also destroy pathogens by stripping the electrons from them. The O_2 molecules cannot pass through our skin. Although the skin is a two-way, semi-permeable membrane, we do not respire through our skin like salamanders do.

We can boost the ozone higher by adding an oxygen bottle to our ozone machine, the higher the percentage of oxygen going through the machine, the higher the level of ozone coming out and going into the bag. Depending on the conditions, great results can be had from just using ambient air, which produces less ozone per liter and requires spending more time in the ozone bag to get the job done. When I bought my first machine, I used it 2 or 3 times for a few hours each time and didn't notice a difference. I concluded that it wasn't working, so I just put it in the closet and forgot about it for about a year.

I have a friend who is a registered nurse and needed a liver transplant. She stopped by one day and told me she didn't think she would live long enough to receive the transplant. She was going downhill rapidly with many health problems. She said that she wished she could afford to buy an ozone machine, as she had heard so many good things about them.

She heard I had an ozone machine and asked me to ozonize water for her to drink. I did it for her, and she drank about a gallon a day. In 3 months, she called me to let me know her doctor told her she no longer needed a liver transplant, and she actually felt good enough to go back to work. I was astounded with the news, but thought she must have been doing other things in addition to drinking ozonized water.

I didn't hear from her for a while. A couple of months passed, and then I ran into her again. She was looking great. I asked her what she had been doing to get her health back. She said, "Just ozone!" She said she felt better than she had in many years. She had bought her own ozone machine and was spending a few hours a day in the bag. All of her other health problems have disappeared as well.

A short time later, I met a retired fireman who had crippling arthritis so bad he hadn't walked upright in more than 10 years. He had already gone through a couple of angioplasties; his doctor had told him he had several blockages and that one artery was 95 percent blocked. This doctor told him he needed bypass surgery immediately, or he may not live long enough to get back to his car. He said that he had been living in such pain for so long that he didn't care if he lived or died. I could completely relate to his statement.

He said that God must have had a plan for him, because his wife took a different route than normal while driving him home, and they went by a church that had a big sign out front that said "Free Ozone Treatments." He told me that after using an ozone machine for 3 months, he no longer had any blockages and was walking upright without pain for the first time in 10 years.

Hearing these stories from people rekindled my interest in using ozone myself. I still wasn't sure how beneficial the treatment would be for me, but I was much more excited about trying it for a longer period of time.

I have since used ozone very successfully for many of my health challenges over the past years. The first couple of years I was apprehensive about using it, as I wasn't sure how beneficial it was and was concerned about its overuse. I decided to buy an oxygen blood tester (Oximeter), so I would know when I needed it and to ensure I did not overuse it.

I have found that almost all identified pathogens, such as most fungi, viruses, bacteria, and neoplasms (cancers), metabolize nitrogen and carry a positive charge (+). All healthy cells in our bodies metabolize oxygen and carry a negative electrical charge (-). The ozone is attracted to the pathogens and denatures them. The debris can then be eliminated by the lymph system and other processes of elimination, such as urination, perspiration, respiration, and defecation.

> Note: The above I have taken from my notes from lectures I have heard at different health trade shows and I don't have the source. Note below is from Dr. Humiston after reviewing this chapter February, 2012.
>
> *Change the paragraph about metabolizing nitrogen; I'm not aware that they do that, or that the nitrogen is important. The explanation is: healthy cells respire oxygen and form antioxidants, which protect them from the effects of ozone. Tumor cells, all viruses, fungi and many bacteria do not produce antioxidants, and are easily killed by ozone.*

Cleansing the circulatory system in this manner is just one of the benefits I am aware of with ozone. I believe this has helped me to clear my own blockages. Also, it is my understanding that fungus, mold, and most harmful bacteria cannot live in an oxygen-rich environment. Oxygen assists in healing most forms of sickness and disease as well as accelerating the healing of injuries.

> *Note: Some of my beliefs have been disputed by some medical doctors and I am not claiming I am right; I am just stating what I observed through my own experiences.*

Many sick people have low levels of oxygen in their blood. The night my mother passed away, my sister told me her oxygen blood level dropped to 40 percent. My assumption is that was the effect caused from her lack of energy allowing her to continue to breathe deeply enough to adequately fill her lungs as she was receiving oxygen through the night. When my oxygen level drops to 93 percent and below, I want to know why; and I start doing something to bring it back up. If it continues to drop, I feel this is an indication of a potentially serious health problem, and I do whatever it takes to get it moving in the right direction. Deep breathing is the fastest way to bring up your blood oxygen level.

A normal blood oxygen level for a healthy person is 94–96 percent. I have seen very sick people with an oxygen level from 94–97 percent, which I attribute to the supplemental nutrients they are taking that allow the blood to absorb and carry the oxygen throughout the body. This is a very positive sign, but in itself does not mean they're getting better. There are other things that must be considered.

For the following several years, every time I felt a cold coming on (or if I was just tired and didn't have any energy), I would test my blood and find that my oxygen blood content was low. I would get into my ozone bag and run the machine. I could bring my blood oxygen content up from about 92 percent to 96 percent while sleeping in the bag overnight. I found that 2–3 nights sleeping in the ozone bag and bringing my oxygen blood level up to 98 percent or 99 percent would eliminate all of my cold symptoms, and my energy level would return.

Understanding that most pathogens cannot live in an oxygen rich environment, I started looking for ways to increase my blood oxygen content to help support my immune system. When I first started using ozone I was concerned about over using it and causing some harm to myself. After buying my oximeter (oxygen blood tester), I would wake up every hour or two to recheck my oxygen blood content. It was 20 or 30 nights before I could relax and feel safe sleeping straight through the night without repeating this process several times.

Now that I have used ozone and other types of oxygen therapies for years, I would suggest that anyone who has a serious health problem consider using some form of oxidation therapy for 30 to 90 days straight, depending on the severity of the health issues. As I understand the simplicity of health, so kindly explained to me by two medical doctors, Dr. Humiston and Dr. Hitt, the underlying cause of most diseases is a disturbance of function from some form of pathogen or environmental toxin causing an imbalance of the internal environment. Oxidation therapy, such as ozone and Sodium Chlorite (MMS), addresses the issue of pathogens that break down the immune system. This helps the immune system to function at its optimal potential *(see chapter 21 for a more thorough explanation).*

Another interesting thing I noticed was that before I started using the ozone bag, I had liver spots (or "aging spots") on my hands and arms. I also was getting a lot of skin tags around my neck, under my arms, and between my legs. After spending the night in my ozone bag 20–30 times, my aging spots turned white, and most of my skin tags went away or got smaller. I have not had a skin tag in the past 15 years.

I went approximately 6 years without a cold using ozone in this manner and expected never to have a cold again! At this point in time, I had never needed to spend more than 3–4 nights in the ozone bag to make me feel good again. I was no longer trying to use it on a particularly serious problem like cancer, AIDS, arthritis, or a heart problem. It was all short-term use and was working so well that I felt it was enough to keep my circulatory system clean. Believing I could eat anything without it hurting me, I had allowed my diet to deteriorate. I thought that using ozone and taking other nutrients was enough to keep me from getting sick. Obviously, I was wrong.

In February of 2002, I had a heart attack. I learned that my oxygen blood content was down to 91 percent the first night I had my chest pains. This was the lowest reading I had ever tested for myself. At that time, I would sleep 5–6 hours a night, as I had been feeling very good. The night I had my first heart attack, I slept for 12 straight hours in my ozone bag without waking up once. My blood oxygen level was up to 97 percent, and I felt much better. I expected to see a reading of 98 percent to 99 percent after that many hours in the ozone bag, but I had never started that low before. I figured out that it took 2 hours for each 1 percent increase, so I was right on target compared to all my previous calculations.

The second evening, when I started feeling tightness in my chest, I checked my oxygen blood level again. It was down to 92 percent. Over the following 7 days, I slept 9 to 10 hours a night in my ozone bag. This excessive use of ozone, along with what I breathed from minor leaks at the drawstring around my neck while I slept, had burned my lungs. A small amount doesn't normally bother us, but the accumulation from that many hours a day for several days in a row took its toll. It took a week off the ozone for my lungs to heal. Now I wrap a towel around my neck to absorb any leaks in that area.

I went back to my cardiologist in May to have all of my original tests rerun to compare the difference in heart damage and blockages from when I had had my 3 heart attacks 3 months earlier. The doctor said I should plan on getting an angiogram and an angioplasty at the same time. He felt my condition was very serious. I agreed to have the angiogram, but I didn't want to do the angioplasty at that time. I felt it would make it much more difficult to clear any remaining blockages once the procedure compressed the plaque and calcium deposits in my veins.

In my research of the use of ozone, one of the most remarkable things I have run across is a videotape of a doctor in Germany being interviewed for a news program about using ozone. He stated that *there have been millions of people successfully treated in Germany with ozone without one death or serious negative side effect.* He himself had successfully treated hundreds of patients, including many with AIDS. When asked if he would participate in a double blind study, he said, “Absolutely not!” When asked why not, he said that he knew what would happen to his AIDS patients—most of the AIDS group would die; but with ozone, most of them would live. He asked, “Why would I want to allow many of my patients to die?”

There are only a few states in the United States that have passed laws allowing doctors to use ozone. Most doctors who do use it make it seem complicated and too difficult for the average person to understand. There are many ways we can use ozone that are much easier to learn. I believe that with ozone, I will live an active, pain-free, healthy life, well beyond 100 years of age, and that it is within everyone’s grasp.

Note that this part of my book was written in 2002. Over the past 10 years, I have learned so much more about the benefits of oxygen therapies and the use of Sodium Chlorite (MMS) that I can now imagine living to at least 150 years old. I believe this is possible while maintaining the quality of life that I knew as a young man as well. Now, at age 70, I am feeling better than I did when I was 20 years old.

One television news show recently showed ozone being used in water treatment for washing meat products in the United States, and they claimed this would stop the recent outbreak of botulism, since ozone kills most all harmful bacteria. Another one showed Japanese companies using it for sterilizing all their food handling equipment. I am sure most people remember the Los Angeles Olympics just a few years ago, when all of the European swim teams refused to compete until the Olympic pool was ozonized and demanded that they stop using chlorine due to its harmful side effects. In my opinion, the more people learn about the benefits of ozone and how cheap it is to use, the less dependent the average person will be on medical doctors and drugs. Anyone can learn to use ozone with just a little knowledge, and once we buy it, it is ours for years.

The lack of research and education about ozone therapy that the AMA and the allopathic medical field in the United States as a whole display is quite a testament to the power of the pharmaceutical industry and their influence over the AMA, the FDA, and our government. They are doing all they can to prevent the dissemination of the beneficial effects of ozone with good reason. I am always astounded by how modern medicine can take so long to recognize a beneficial treatment when human life is at stake. Could it be because there is no money to be made from the use of ozone? As long as the lobbyists can convince our representatives in Washington, D.C., that anything outside of mainstream medicine is dangerous, fraudulent, or useless, the United States will continue to have the most expensive, and worst, health care of all developed countries in the world. (This excludes emergency medicine, of which we no doubt have the best in the world.)

13 major effects of ozone on the human body, compiled by Dr. Frank Shallenberger, MD, are listed below with brief explanations:

1) Ozone stimulates the production of white blood cells. These cells protect the body from viruses, bacteria, fungi, and cancer. Deprived of oxygen, these cells malfunction. They fail to eliminate invaders and even turn against normal, healthy cells (allergic reactions). Ozone significantly raises oxygen levels in the blood for long periods after ozone administration; as a result.

2) Interferon levels are significantly increased. Interferons are globular proteins that orchestrate every aspect of the

immune system. Some interferons are produced by cells infected by viruses. These interferons, adjacent to healthy cells, are more likely to spread infection; in turn, they are rendered non-permissive host cells. In other words, they inhibit viral replication. Other interferons are produced in the muscles, connective tissue, and by white blood cells.

Ozone can elevate levels of gamma interferon by 400–900 percent. Gamma interferon is involved in the control of phagocytic cells that engulf and kill pathogens and abnormal cells. Interferons are FDA approved for the treatment of chronic hepatitis B and C, genital warts (caused by papillomavirus), hairy-cell leukemia, Kaposi's sarcoma, relapsing-remitting multiple sclerosis, and chronic granulomatous disease, and are currently in clinical trials for throat warts (caused by papillomavirus), HIV infection, chronic myelogenous leukemia, leukemia, non-Hodgkin's lymphoma, colon tumors, kidney tumors, bladder cancer, malignant melanoma, basal cell carcinoma, and leishmaniasis.

3) Ozone stimulates the production of tumor necrosis factor (TNF). TNF is produced by the body when a tumor is growing. The greater the mass of the tumor, the more tumor necrosis factor is produced (up to a point). When a tumor metastastasizes, cancer cells break off and are carried away by the blood and lymph system. This allows the tumor to take up residence elsewhere in the body or, in other words, distribute its forces. These lone cancer cells have little chance of growing in the levels of TNF produced

to inhibit the original tumor. When the tumor is removed surgically, TNF levels drop dramatically and new tumors emerge from seemingly healthy tissue.

4) Ozone stimulates the secretion of interleukin-2 (IL-2). IL-2 is one of the cornerstones of the immune system. It is secreted by T-helpers. In a process known as auto-stimulation, IL-2 binds to a receptor on the T-helper and causes it to produce more IL-2. Its main duty is to induce lymphocytes to differentiate and proliferate, yielding more T-helpers, T-suppressors, cytotoxic Ts, and T-memory cells.

5) Low concentrations of ozone kill most bacteria. The metabolism of most bacteria is, on average, 1/17th as efficient as our own. Because of this, most cannot afford to produce disposable antioxidant enzymes such as catalase; thus, very few types of bacteria can live in an environment composed of more than 2 percent ozone.

6) Ozone is effective against all types of fungi. This includes systemic *Candida albicans*, athlete's foot, molds, mildews, yeasts, and even mushrooms.

7) Ozone fights viruses in a variety of ways. One is going after viral particles directly. The part of the virus most sensitive to oxidation is the reproductive structure that allows viruses to enter cells. When this structure is inactivated, the virus is essentially "dead." Cells already infected have a natural weakness to ozone. Due to the metabolic burden of the infection, the cells can no longer produce the enzymes necessary to deal with the ozone and repair the cell.

8) Ozone is antineoplastic. This means that ozone inhibits the growth of new tissue, because rapidly dividing cells shift their priorities away from producing the enzymes needed to protect themselves from the ozone. Cancer cells are rapidly dividing cells and are inhibited by ozone.

9) Ozone oxidizes arterial plaque. It breaks down the main plaque involved in arteriosclerosis. This means ozone has a tendency to clear blockages of large and even smaller vessels. This allows for better tissue oxygenation in deficient organs.

10) Ozone increases the flexibility and elasticity of red blood cells. Under a microscope, a red blood cell looks like a disc. They pick up oxygen in the capillaries of the lungs and distribute it to every cell of the body. The cell discs stretch out into the shape of an oval or umbrella to aid their passage through the tiny capillaries; this makes the exchange of oxygen and other nutrients more efficient. Higher red blood cell flexibility allows oxygen levels to stay elevated for days, even weeks, after treatment with ozone.

11) Ozone accelerates the citric acid cycle. Also known as the Krebs cycle or TCA cycle, this is a very important step in the glycolysis of carbohydrates for energy that takes place in the mitochondria of the cell. Most of the energy stored in glucose (sugar) is converted in this pathway. 10–15 drops of a 50 percent citric acid solution in 4–6 ounces of water will introduce this energy into your body—and it may be even more beneficial if you ozonate the water prior to drinking it.

12) Ozone makes the antioxidant enzyme system more efficient.

13) Ozone degrades petrochemicals. These chemicals place potentially great burden on the immune system. They also worsen (and even cause) allergies and are detrimental to our long-term health.

While in Costa Rica in 1996, I met a Cuban doctor who told me AIDS has been successfully treated with ozone for many years. She also told me she had used it many times for clearing blockages in the circulatory system, dramatically reducing heart disease. She said it is the least expensive form of treatment for many, if not most, diseases and had no serious side effects other than the occasional headache. Now and then, someone might "burn" his or her lungs if he or she breathes it, but that is rare. In a week or two, the lungs will heal themselves with no lasting, harmful side effects in most cases.

I wasn't sure how much of her story I could really believe, since at that time I still struggled with *wanting* to believe that our government would not withhold information about the benefit and use of ozone unless there was a downside. In 2006, when I met Dr. William Hitt and Dr. John Humiston working in Tijuana, Mexico, they told me they would rather work in Mexico for a dime on the dollar of what they could make working in the United States. Why? Because they could treat their patients as their conscience dictated and had the freedom to use ozone there. That woke me up to the reality of the collusion between the FDA and the pharmaceutical industry.

Dr. Hitt was nearly 80 years old at the time and had been working in Mexico for almost 30 years, using ozone very successfully for many forms of disease.

The Cuban doctor told me that Cuba has more prostitutes per capita than any place in the world that she was aware of. They are all required to carry a working permit or go to jail. They are also required to have a weekly physical examination to check for AIDS and all the other venereal diseases. If they are found to be HIV positive or have any form of venereal disease, they are taken off the street and put into a sanitarium for treatment. Treatment with ozone eliminates most AIDS and venereal diseases within 2 weeks. Even the most difficult cases usually respond well to ozone, and they never have to resort to antibiotics for treatment.

Gary Forester, a naturopathic doctor from Texas who was living in Costa Rica at that time, was allowing two female doctors from Cuba to live in his home while they were on vacation, and they confirmed what I had been previously told by another Cuban doctor a couple of years earlier.

Ozone and Arthritis

Cartilage is a living tissue made up of dense connective tissue. Cartilage is classified in 3 types—elastic cartilage, hyaline cartilage, and fibrocartilage—which differ in the relative amounts of these 3 main components.

A. Cartilage is found in many areas in the body, including the articular surface of the bones, the rib cage, the ear, the nose, the bronchial tubes, and the intervertebral disks. Its mechanical properties are intermediate between bone and dense connective tissue like tendon.

B. Unlike other connective tissues, cartilage does not contain blood vessels. The chondrocytes are fed by diffusion, helped by the pumping action generated by compression of the articular cartilage or flexion of the elastic cartilage. Thus, compared to other connective tissues, cartilage grows and repairs more slowly.

C. Rheumatoid arthritis is an autoimmune disease that causes chronic inflammation of the joints. Rheumatoid arthritis can also cause inflammation of the tissue around the joints, as well as in other organs in the body. A joint is where two bones meet to allow movement of body parts. *Arthritis* means "joint inflammation." The joint inflammation of rheumatoid arthritis causes swelling, pain, stiffness, and redness in the joints. The inflammation of rheumatoid disease can also occur in tissues around the joints, such as the tendons, ligaments, and muscles.

In some people with rheumatoid arthritis, chronic inflammation leads to the destruction of the cartilage, bone, and ligaments, causing deformity of the joints. Damage to the joints can occur early in the disease and be progressive. Moreover, studies have shown that the progressive damage to the joints does not necessarily correlate with the degree of pain, stiffness, or swelling present in the joints. Rheumatoid arthritis is a common rheumatic disease, affecting 1,000,000 people in the United States.

From several doctors I have heard lecture at health trade shows, I believe that rheumatoid arthritis in many cases can be linked to a long-term imbalance in our blood pH. Because the body's blood must maintain a pH of 7.35 (± 0.2 pH), and most of the things we eat, drink, and breathe produce acid, the body steals calcium from our bones in order to neutralize the acid and maintain balance.

I prefer an organically grown food source calcium with 1/3 calcium and 2/3 magnesium along with the many other nano-components that science has no knowledge of at this time. Rock source calcium is most commonly sold at health food stores because it is much less expensive and it meets the FDA's labeling standards even though the body cannot properly assimilate most of it.

The body's ideal blood pH is 7.35, according to Nutripathic, Dr. Sal D'Onofrio. Maximum blood oxygen content is achieved at

7.4 pH. The problem is that once the body uses the calcium from bones and teeth to rebalance the blood pH, it redeposits it into the soft tissue and joints. Your bones and tissues become calcium deficient. The body requires a rebalancing of calcium and magnesium through diet and digestion.

This type of calcium remnant is an element highly susceptible to oxidation by ozone. Ozone breaks down the arthritic calcium; it is not a complete molecule, which allows it to be carried off as waste. Since cells do not maintain it, it is not replaced. This leaves normal cartilage and bone unharmed. In fact, ozone actually strengthens bone and cartilage by oxidizing the blockage in the blood vessels supplying the bone, allowing increased nutrients to flow through.

In a study done in Havana, Cuba, 60 patients with osteoarthritis were given one intramuscular injection of ozone per week for a total of 10 weeks. Of the 60 patients, painful symptoms returned in only 4 patients after 2 months, while 93.3 percent remained pain free. This has been proven to be a safe, easily applied, and low-cost therapy. Most were pain free after the first several ozone treatments. In almost everyone, the inflammation of the joints and restoration of normal joint movement was over 90 percent.

In 1990, there was another study in Cuba in which 233 patients suffering from arthritis—progressive degeneration of cartilage in the spine, knees, and other joints—were given 20 intramuscular injections of ozone over a period of 30 days. Of that number, 208 patients (89 percent) reported improvement, and only 2 stated they had no relief.

The presence of ozone causes white blood cells to reproduce at a much faster rate. Ozone acts like a free radical, since O_3 is electron deficient; that is, it is looking for electrons. The pathogenic organisms that metabolize nitrogen and are electron rich become the electron donors. The cancer cells or others that are nitrogen metabolizers are thus destroyed, while the white blood cells (immune cells) increase.

Research shows tumor cells shrink when subjected to ozone. Tumor cells have a high rate of glucose uptake and lactic acid production in an oxygen-rich environment. This implies they are anaerobic and therefore only $1/17^{th}$ as efficient as aerobic cells. Ozone is harmless to most healthy cells. In fact, ozone even makes the antioxidant enzyme systems of normal cells more efficient.

The best-known American doctor that I am aware of who uses ozone is Dr. Kurt W. Donsbach, founder of the Hospital Santa Monica in Mexico, a holistic health care facility. He has treated thousands of cancer patients with ozone via humidified rectal insufflation. In a letter to Nathaniel Altman, author of *Oxygen Healing Therapies*, Dr. Donsbach reports, "Approximately 70 percent of our patients are alive, 3 years after their first visit to our facility. Some are cured, some are in remission, and some are slowly dying. However, very few of these patients had more than months to live according to their doctors when they arrived. But what kind of statistics are these? We see a significant percentage of our patients become totally and completely cured as documented by medical diagnostic standards." (I obtained written permission to quote this from his book.)

Ozone is not always successful, but its success rate is much higher than traditional treatments. It is also very important to consider that its adverse side effect rate is only 0.000005 per application, which is far lower than any other drug or form of treatment. Ozone usually reduces the side effects of traditional therapies, most of which poison the body in an attempt to kill the tumor.

Ozone works incredibly well on gangrene. Even in the worst cases, there is hope with ozone and other oxidative forms of treatment. There is very little dispute over the best way to use ozone in this situation. Most physicians agree that the bagging method is far superior. The affected limb is put inside a bag, which is then inflated with ozone.

The type of ozone bag I recommend is double-stitched cotton sailcloth; it has to be custom made (I don't know of a store that sells them). Because ozone is so corrosive, I don't recommend using plastic, as it could break down and harmful contaminants could be absorbed through the skin into your blood along with the ozone.

When used in this way, ozone has a remarkable ability to increase the local blood supply. Even when the whole body is bagged, a flushing of the skin is noticeable. This is the basic problem in gangrene: not enough oxygenated fresh blood is getting to the area. Of course, this is not the underlying cause, but increasing the local blood supply can save the limb in most cases.

There are two main causes of gangrene: either blood can't get to the area or it can't get away. In patients suffering from diabetes, not enough blood is getting to the area because too much is being diverted to the muscles and brain. Gangrene is often caused by blockage in an artery carrying blood to the tissue. This is the same blockage involved in angina attacks and arteriosclerosis, and I believe ozone is very effective in clearing these blockages. I have talked to many doctors as well as many people that use ozone who claim this is true; it has worked on my own arterial blockages. I will admit I have talked to a few doctors that say this is not an accurate statement. I often do many things at the same time so I can't say beyond a doubt that ozone is a major part of clearing my blockages but I was using ozone along with other types of chelation and the blockages went away.

Ozone's ability to dramatically increase blood oxygen is something no medication can do. It may not work 100 percent of the time for others, but so far it has worked 100 percent of the time with my health problems. Since it is so inexpensive, safe, and easy to use, it seems to me that this is a good place to start for those who want to learn to help themselves.

For more information, see the International Ozone Association's website: www.int-ozone-assoc.org/ioaweb2.html.

Also, an informative book that may give you a unique look into the future of alternative health care is *God Wants You to Be Rich*, by Paul Zane Pilzer. The author is an economist who believes our world is full of limitless wealth and resources. Dr. Pilzer says that we can live well beyond 100 years if we take responsibility for our own health. He is also one of the economists who guided President Reagan through Reaganomics. He successfully predicted the computer boom during the 1980s and the Internet boom in the 1990s. He now predicts that in the next 10 years, alternative health care will be the next trillion-dollar industry. He believes it will outperform all other industries in this country.

I believe this as well, because the United States of America's health care system is broken, and everyone knows it. The cost of our health care is nearly that of the rest of the world combined, and at a lecture I heard a doctor recently say we are now rated 47th in *quality* of health care, with the exception of emergency medicine. He also said that there are over 300,000 lawsuits against large pharmaceutical companies and other medical malpractice suits. In addition, there are 320,000 lawsuits pending against the FDA and different state laws regarding alternative health. This industry is collapsing under its own greedy weight as more and more people are waking up to the corruption in our government that allows FDA personnel to moonlight for the pharmaceutical industry.

In conclusion, my many years of using ozone have benefited me a great deal and reversed many of my health issues. The use of ozone has given me a very good understanding of oxidative therapies and this knowledge, along with my personal use and benefit, allowed me to appreciate Sodium Chlorite (MMS) as well. Meeting Jim Humble in Mexico in February of 1997 opened my eyes to just how simple health can be. Jim explained how Sodium Chlorite (MMS) oxidizes pathogens and environmental toxins in a way similar to ozone without harming the friendly flora needed for digestion. This made perfect sense to me, and I started using it with fantastic success—even for many things that were not practical for ozone use.

I highly support Jim Humble's work; he is a true humanitarian who has made a very valuable contribution and works tirelessly spreading the word about the many benefits of Sodium Chlorite (MMS).

I have used oxidative therapies for nearly 20 years now, and I have spoken to thousands of people who have successfully used some form of oxidation in restoring their health. Today there are many books about the benefits of oxidation, and I have never read about anyone dying from its use. To my knowledge, there never has been a proven death from the use of oxidative therapies.

Understanding oxidative therapies, through what I have read and the many benefits that I have received, has made me realize that health can be just that simple. Adding more oxygen to your blood any way you can will help you make *Your Health Your Choice.*

CHAPTER 4

Magnetic Therapy

Magnetic and oxidative therapies are the two most important therapies I have studied and used to reverse many of my health issues. To me, this has made the difference between living and dying, not to mention the rapid reduction in pain and suffering. They are also very inexpensive. Once we buy the few things we need, they're ours for life.

Magnet therapy is not accepted as a medical practice by the vast majority of allopathic mainstream doctors in this country, but I assure you, it works. Most countries around the world use it to varying degrees. In the Far East, most drugstores sell magnets like we sell aspirin. While aspirin only reduces pain and does little to nothing to help accelerate the healing, magnets do both.

There are more and more electromagnetic healing devices being patented and manufactured all the time that work very well. They sell for thousands of dollars and require a doctor's prescription to even use them; they are restricted for sale to doctors only. For me, this is just more proof of collusion between the FDA and the pharmaceutical industry as this unconscionable scam continues to be perpetrated on us, the citizens of the United States. I have received incredible benefit from the use of inexpensive magnets by following the advice of a few doctors who have been good enough to teach me how to best deal with my own health issues. I could write a whole book on it.

Magnetic energy has been used for healing at least as far back as recorded history. The Egyptians, Chinese, and Greeks have recorded its use for thousands of years. Modern science has established that a magnetic energy field moves through all living matter. These fields, when in sync with the earth's field, will have a positive effect on all living things at the cellular level, thus influencing our mental and physical welfare. In recent years, widespread public acceptance has turned magnetic therapy into a $5 billion a year world market.

Because there is a definite difference in effect from positive and negative fields, it is very important to know where to place the positive pole and the length of time it can safely be applied. The positive field triggers a false injury crisis, like an acupuncture needle, and the body responds by sending its reserve healing energy to the area to fight the battle or repair damage. It is my understanding that after a short time, the body eventually realizes it has been tricked when a positive magnetic field is used, and the mind recalls its defense forces just like an army. One can use the negative pole of a magnet continuously for hours, but never use the positive side for more than 20 minutes at a time unless supervised by a specialist. The only one I personally know and would trust with the use of the positive field is Dr. Dean Bonlie, a Canadian dentist who now lives in Las Vegas.

By stimulating the magnetic fields of our cells, we can reduce pain and anxiety and accelerate healing by several times the normal rate.

Following is a list of benefits that I have personally received from magnetic therapy from treating myself with inexpensive individual magnets as well as sleeping on an under-the-mattress magnetic pad:

- Prostate issues overcome.
- Ruptured disk in my neck healed: range of motion increased from 10 percent to 15 percent to full range of

motion within 3 months, using a large magnet on my neck. This was after more than 2 years of no progress from the therapy prescribed by several specialists, medical doctors, and therapists. The State of Nevada paid thousands of dollars for little to no result, as I was injured on the job at a large fire. I was told to learn to live with it and that it would not get better.

- Degenerated lower back disks that caused a great deal of pain, healed in a few months.
- Cartilage in my right knee healed in a few months.
- Muscle in my left leg revitalized and healed from a 25-year-old horseback riding injury.
- Heart damage as the result of 3 heart attacks, repaired.
- Broken bones healed in 2 weeks, as opposed to the "normal" 6 weeks.
- Severely sprained ankle mended sufficiently to walk on within 24 hours.
- Several mashed fingers healed without loss of the fingernail within 3 days.
- A torn rotator cuff that had been hurting me for 2 years was healed in 2 days.
- Elbow injury healed.
- Gum infection resolved. Pain was dramatically reduced within a few minutes, and symptoms of the infection were gone within a few days.
- Stopped many nose bleeds quickly by using a 4 x 6 x 1 inch magnet like a cold pack on the back of my neck.

- Torn hamstring: I was fully functional after one week of using magnets, and the bruising was gone as well.

The picture below was taken December 4, 2005. The injury was from playing ping pong in China; I slipped and tore my hamstring muscle. It would have been much worse, but I did have a 4 inch x 4 inch x ¼ inch magnet with me, and I placed it in a critical place within an hour.

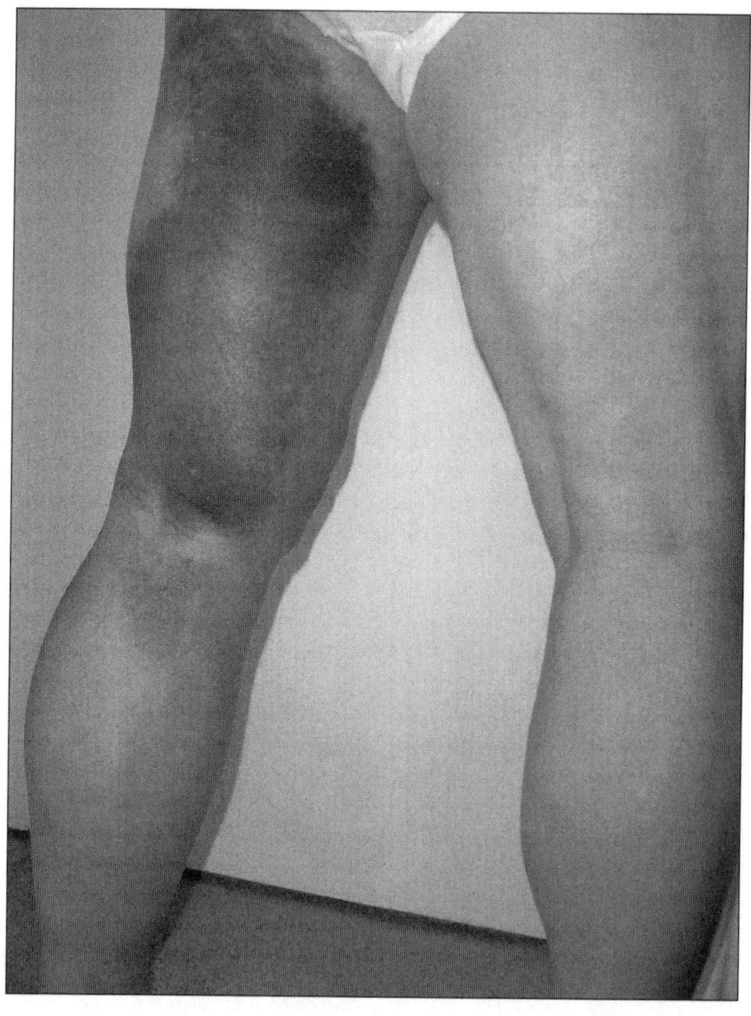

The two pictures below were taken after my return home; and they show how I used the magnets.

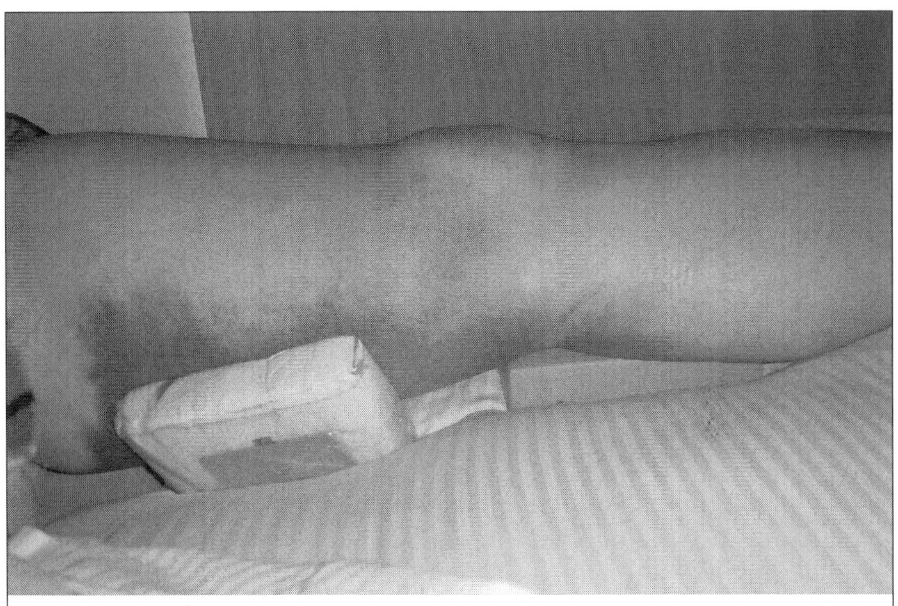

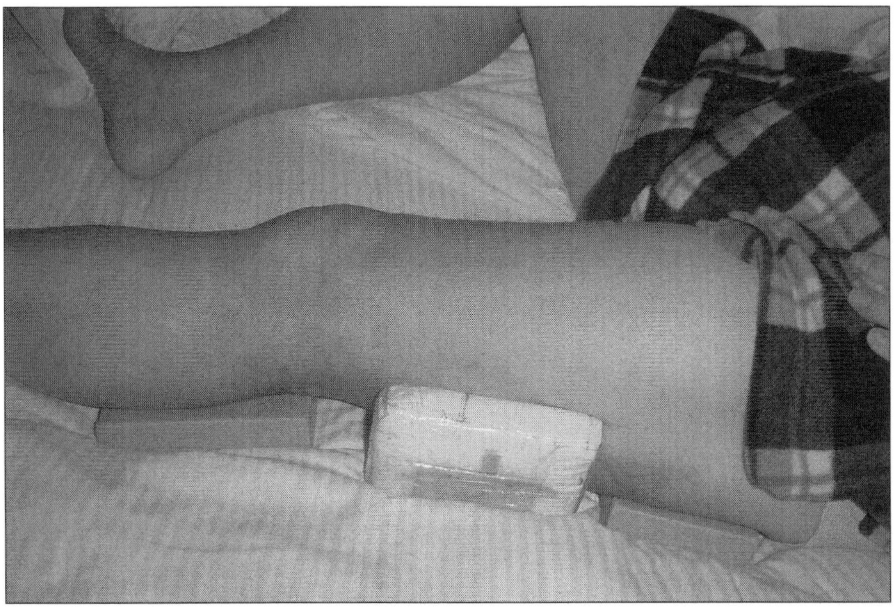

The following picture was taken later after using four 4 x 6 x 1 inch magnets for just one day.

The below photo shows the padded metal device I made to hold the magnets on each side of my leg. In 1992, I had used the magnets covered in white on each side of my knee when I overcame my knee injury. I never received the operation doctors wanted to do on me.

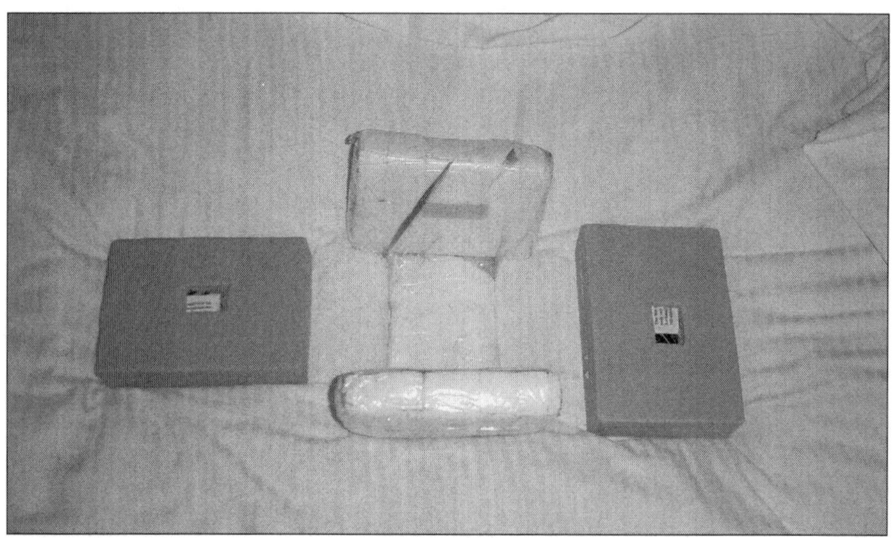

The larger and more powerful the magnet, the faster I saw the benefit. The magnet I use most is 4 x 6 x 1 inches and weighs about 5 pounds. Nearly all the benefits I have received have been from the bio-north (negative) pole field only, especially during the first 24 hours of a new injury. On older injuries, I have received some incredible benefits from the use of the positive field, but do not use it for more than 20 minutes at a time.

I know there are many acupuncturists who use very small magnets in lieu of needles and get great results. Years ago, because of the fear of HIV and hepatitis B and C being spread with needles, many clinics decided to play it safe and switch to magnets so they would not lose business. Acupuncturists quickly adapted to the use of magnets and found they were getting results that were just as good; many continue to use them today.

I personally haven't taken the time to try to learn the subtleties of using magnets the way many specialists have. I just wanted the pain to go away, now. The accelerated healing of any injury or health issue is an added benefit. I choose to use a large magnet wherever the pain is, and I get fantastic results with it.

Warnings:

- Never use a magnet on someone with a pacemaker or a defibrillator.
- Make sure you learn the difference between the bio-magnetic, north pole and the north pole that is marked for industrial use. (The bio-north pole is the south-seeking pole of all magnets.) Your life could depend on it.
- I have been advised to state a warning against magnet use for anyone who is pregnant or for a child under 5 years old. I don't know why this could be a problem, but because a close friend who is a doctor suggested this; I feel it should be mentioned.

It is important to understand the different effects of the negative (-) bio-north pole and the positive (+) bio-south pole. ("Bio" means "having to do with the body" and the (-) bio-north pole is the south-seeking pole of all magnets.)
Difference between the bio-magnetic and the magnetic north pole:

All references made in this chapter are to the use of bio-marked magnets. Any time you are in doubt of the direction your magnet is to be used, just tie a string around it and let it hang down or dangle. When it stops turning, the south-seeking pole is the bio-north pole and is the side that should face your body most of the time. But when treating the front part of the body, use the bio-south pole to keep consistent with the earth's magnetic field. This is what I have been taught, and I follow it exactly most of the time. But when I treat the front of my body with the South Pole, I never do it without a second magnet on the back side with the north pole facing toward my body. The best results are obtained when you use magnets that support the earth's magnetic field. In the northern hemisphere, we receive exposure to a magnetic field going from sky to the earth. If you customarily sleep on your back or side, you will use the negative, bio-north pole facing your back or sides.

The energy needs to be used as required by the circumstance of an injury or illness. When you need to use multiple magnets to cover a large area with the same polarity, they need to be kept close together, as there will be a bleed-through from the opposing pole when they're too far apart. There is so much to know about this subject that I cannot cover it all in this chapter. Much of the information in many books on magnet therapy is wrong. My personal recommendation is to contact the Magnetico Company at www.magnetico.com, or call them at 800-265-1119. Their website has information that I completely trust. Their products can be used safely without spending the many thousands of dollars and many years that I have to educate myself in the proper use and benefits of magnet energy.

Some of the body's pains can be increased with a positive magnetic influence. Sleeping on a pure negative magnetic field on a properly designed bed can give your body's energy a boost that can restore health and vitality. This will help balance the harmful effects of the 60-cycle electromagnetic fields that we are exposed to every day. Thousands of people have experienced reduction or total elimination of pain when sleeping on such a mattress. It has made a definite improvement in my life.

The reason I stress the pure field is that if two negative magnets are placed close together, they repel each other. There will always be a gap between them, and in that gap there will be a positive (+) spike. It will extend above the top of the negative sides of the two magnets. The height reached depends on the distance between the magnets. The key points in deciding which mattress to buy are the design and spacing of the magnets and the placement of the magnets under the mattress. It is necessary to maintain adequate space above the top of the positive peaks rising from between the magnets on the magnetic pad.

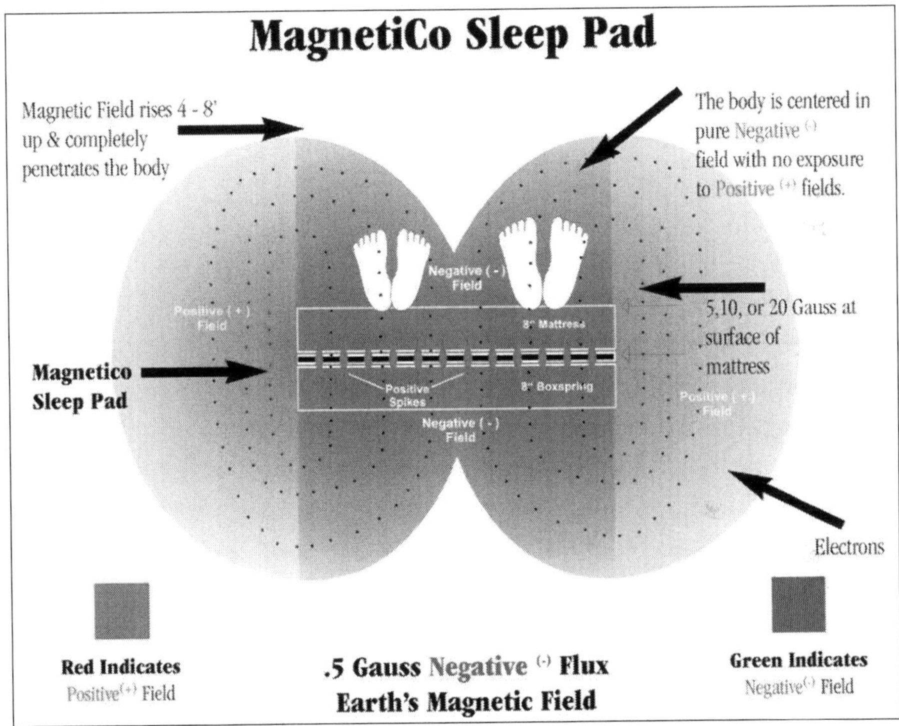

The above diagram was provided by Dr. Dean Bonlie to better illustrate how the earth's magnetic energy flows. He has discovered something very interesting about it, and I believe that few others, if any, have ever figured out just how this energy flows.

Electromagnetic fields are the energy of life, and they come naturally from our brain. All of our cells carry a charge—not just the brain. All of our bodily functions are controlled and driven by electromagnetic energy. Every thought or action or involuntary action and responses are 100 percent dependent on this energy.

The frequencies emitted by the brain are specific for resonance and messaging as well as muscle control. 60-cycle frequency, which most electrical power comes in, will interfere with our natural frequencies.

The body's biochemistry process is actually controlled and governed by the electromagnetic field our body generates. By enhancing that field, we can reduce pain, anxiety and accelerate healing by several times the normal rate. When you consider that every cell in your body is electromagnetic and depends on interaction between them (each organ has a different vibrational frequency), it starts to make sense that you can treat your body with magnetic energy. I view each of our bodies as an orchestra; when these frequencies are in harmony, what we hear is beautiful music, and our health becomes optimal. If these harmonious frequencies are sustained, they work synergistically to maximize both mental and physical health. We are energy beings: we are .9999-plus percent space held together by the energy electrons create as they spin around atomic nuclei. The energy that holds our cells together is the same type of energy that makes all bodily cells. By increasing magnetic energy, we increase electrons' orbital velocity. This increases their energy state and increases the cells' ability to repair and replicate faster.

To help me remember how to use my magnets, I associate the color blue with the cold of the North Pole, which is at the negative mark (-) on many properly marked magnets. Even though the earth's South Pole is just as cold as the North Pole, I think of the positive (+) or South Pole as hot and associate it with the color red. I use a magnet the same way I use hot and cold packs on an injury, only the magnets are far more effective. This lengthy explanation may not make sense to you right now, but everyone needs to understand that some magnets are only marked with the signs for negative and positive, while a few manufacturers indicate the poles by painting one side red or blue and leaving the other unpainted. It is rare to find a manufacturer that states clearly which side is which. I have found more times than not that magnets come marked for industrial use and that they mark the polarity incorrectly. It is very important to understand this before attempting to utilize magnetic energy for healing.

For all new injuries, I use only the negative (-), north pole for the first 24 hours. After that, I alternate north and south poles every 20 minutes. My broken ribs were healed in 10 days when I was in Costa Rica. The pain was gone in less than a month. The medical doctor who took the X-rays had said that it would take 6 weeks to heal and up to 6 months for the pain to go away.

Here is an experiment you can do yourself: take two 4 x 6 x 1 inch magnets and place a glass of whole milk on each of them—one on the positive side and one on the negative side. Put them about 3 feet apart to avoid overlapping fields. Put a third glass of whole milk on the counter as a control glass. In my experiment, the milk on the positive side was definitely spoiled and had an odor much faster than either of the other two. By the third day, I threw away the control glass, as it had an odor as well. A week later, the glass sitting on the negative side still smelled fresh. I didn't try to drink it, since I couldn't say for sure that it was bacteria free, but its lack of odor was impressive. (If you do this experiment, do not use fat-free milk, as its odors are not as noticeable.)

I felt that this supported what I had read: that the negative field retarded bacterial growth, and the positive field enhances bacterial growth. When work on building something with wood, I frequently get a splinter and seldom take time to pull it out or clean and wrap it. I know from several firsthand experiences that when I put a small neodymium magnet with its negative side to the infected finger, the throbbing and pain go away quickly and the infection is gone in a day or two.

I am not recommending that anyone do some of the things I have done to myself without getting a lot more information than I am able to put in this book. When I started writing, I had just finished a magnetic therapy certification course, and I am still learning and seeking information about many benefits of magnetic energy 20 years later. I have also listened to many doctors lecture on the subject and attended several 2 and 3 day seminars. Even after reading over a dozen books on the subject, I still have so much more to learn about using magnets and their many benefits.

According to Dr. DeHann, magnets have been used successfully in medical therapy for humans and animals for hundreds of years, particularly for the treatment of osteoarthritis. Experiments at Loma Linda University in California, the Massachusetts Institute of Technology, and several universities in Europe have shown that magnetic devices improve blood flow to damaged tissues, speeding the healing process. Magnetism, the doctor writes, helps to order and align tissue salts in damaged cells. Electromagnetic stimulation gets the damaged tissues' fluids flowing again, helping to speed the elimination of waste products, reduce swelling, and restore normal function.

This dramatically supports what I stated a few pages earlier about suppressed knowledge. This should be taught to every child in our school system and the mainstream media should make the benefits of magnetic healing and other forms of energy healing public knowledge. I have heard nothing from the mainstream media since this information was first released many years ago.

For people who suffer from back and neck pain, magnets can ease the pain and swelling. Once I started using magnetic therapy, I got immediate relief from the pain of the ruptured disk in my neck. I also noticed a dramatic improvement each day in my range of motion; I was able to do stretching exercises that I was not able to do before. As I improved, I noticed less and less improvement with the magnetic therapy treatment because I was getting better. The more you need the benefit, the more benefit you notice. When you start healing, you don't notice the daily improvement as much.

The therapy can benefit patients with many painful health problems such as osteoporosis, arthritis, ruptured or deteriorated disks, and damaged cartilage. Most people accept their doctor's word that there is nothing that can be done for them and settle for using medication to hide the pain in their effort to live a pain-free life. I have been there with all of the above. Now, when I have any sign of pain, I know just what to do. I use one of the many sizes of magnets I have bought over the years for different specific uses, and I have never been disappointed in the results. I love feeling 20 years old once again and being pain free.

I had a bone scan done several years ago, and it showed that I was in the normal range for my age. I requested the doctor explain in more detail. He said that I didn't have any signs of osteoporosis! I asked if that meant I had no bone loss. He replied, "Of course there's bone loss, but you are in the normal range for your age." He said that 34 percent loss was normal! I said that this was not acceptable and asked what I could do about it. He told me that there was nothing I could do; it was just a part of growing old.

This motivated me to start looking into the cause of osteoporosis, and I found that nearly all of us are experiencing bone loss. The body must maintain a blood pH of 7.35 (± 0.2). Since most of the things we eat, drink, even breathe (especially as we exercise), cause us to produce even more acid, the body must steal calcium from the bones in order to neutralize the acid and maintain a balanced pH. This lack of calcium in the blood and acidic diet can be a cause of osteoporosis.

Once I understood what caused the problem, I started asking many doctors and alternative health care professionals what to do about it and soon found what worked for me. About this time, I bought one of Dr. Bonlie's magnetic mattresses. I then supplemented my diet with Mobil-Ease and Herbal CA. Mobil-Ease is made by Prevail, and it is an enzyme-based nutritional product that works together with the Herbal CA to restore bone. Herbal CA is a plant-based calcium made from many different types of herbs by Nature's Sunshine Company. Although it is a very good product, I no longer use the Herbal CA with Mobil-Ease. I use Bone Support by A2Z Health Products instead, because it is 100 percent bioavailable and it also rejuvenates the bones.

When I started the above regimen in 1992, all of my teeth were loose, as I had a substantial amount of bone loss at this time in my life. I had lost a couple of them, and many of my remaining teeth were quite loose. I felt certain they would all fall out within 2–3 years; however, within 3 months, all of my teeth had tightened up a lot, as the bone density was restored. I went back to the doctor, and he reran a bone scan with the same machine 2 years after I started using these supplements and sleeping on the magnetic mattress. I had 105 percent of the bone density of a 20 year old.

I didn't know at the time that magnetism could stop bone loss. For several years, I was giving all the credit to just the supplements until I heard Dr. Bonlie lecture on his magnetic sleep pad at a trade show. This was about the 10th time I had heard him. Finally, the light came on in my head. Reversing the bone density loss was not just the nutritional supplements I was taking. He mentioned that stopping bone loss is one of the important features of sleeping on an increased magnetic field. I can't say for sure which played the most important part for me, but I feel it was the combination of the nutritional supplements and the magnetic energy that allowed the amazing accelerated reversal of bone loss. In addition, the arthritis pain in my back was completely relieved along with the pain from the ruptured disk in my neck. The ruptured disk shrank to the point that I no longer even noticed any discomfort at all.

I read recently in a magazine that the famous actor Anthony Hopkins strongly endorses magnets for lower and upper back pain relief. He had shoulder pain for years; all other options were eliminated, yet no relief was found. "They're the answer to my prayers!" exclaimed Mr. Hopkins.

Below I list a number of personal stories about the benefits I have received from the use of magnets. I wrote most of them when they happened. I begin with my first dramatic experience because I have a point that will become apparent later.

Prostatitis and Prostate Cancer

Chronic prostatitis that eventually became cancer plagued me for over 10 years. All the while, I believed that doctors had the final word on the subject. Because of my lack of knowledge concerning my own health issues, prostate cancer was one of the most difficult things to overcome. Three different urologists had me take antibiotics for months at a time; the last cycle lasted a whole year without a break and was of no permanent help. I tried everything I could find at the time but found only temporary relief.

This was the most serious health issue I had faced at the time I was diagnosed. I believed that if a doctor couldn't heal me, my life was over; I had no confidence in my ability to make a difference in my own health. Today, I realize there are many ways to address all forms of cancer, and that it is nothing to fear. I look at any new health issue as just another opportunity to learn more about what I can do for myself to reverse whatever the new condition may be. Our lack of knowledge and belief that health is complicated beyond our ability to understand causes fear and often prevents us from taking the first step in making our health our choice. The first step is educating ourselves and learning about the increasing number of people who have been successful in reversing their health challenges.

In 1991, I met Dr. Bonlie, who uses magnetic therapy extensively in his research and treatment. Dr. Bonlie gave me a very powerful 4 x 6 x 1 inch ceramic magnet and told me to sit on its bio-north pole (-) every time I watched television, drove, or sat down for any reason. In one month, most of the prostate symptoms were gone, and within 3 months, all the symptoms were completely gone. I continued to use it for 3 more months, and I have not had a problem with prostatitis for many years. My PSA test dropped from 77 to 7 within the first 3 months, which is an amazing reduction; not long after that, I had it checked again. It was less than 1, a very healthy number. The doctor explained that the magnet did not cure me, as only our body can do that, but it helped to provide the energy my body needed to do the job more efficiently.

I want to point out that I have been experiencing some minor noticeable return of the symptoms of this issue starting around 2009. It has not been much of a concern to date, as I seldom even remember to use a magnet. I have been using an electronic heat probe that I insert rectally. The temperature goes up to 114 degrees Fahrenheit. I understand that cancer cannot survive a temperature above 106 degrees. I should use this probe 2 times a day, morning and night, every day. Because the symptoms are so minor, I often forget to use it, and I find myself using it just a few times a week. It does seem to be having a beneficial effect, but it is too soon for me to say for sure at this point. I know so many ways to address cancer at this point in my education that I have no concerns about this becoming serious. I am always looking forward to finding new and better ways to help my body heal itself. I find myself thankful when I have a health issue, as it motivates me to continue learning more ways to address each issue. I feel our future in medicine is exciting as I learn more about the use of energy. I feel that soon we will all be able to manifest our health energetically and everyone will realize just how simple health can be.

Dr. Bonlie has had incredible success in his research using magnetic energy to relieve pain and accelerate healing. In several cases, he has been able to get paraplegic patients up and walking. I have received so many benefits using magnets; I always carry a small magnet with me in case of an emergency. I have used it many times to test manufacturers' mattresses and other products. Dr. Bonlie's mattress is the only one that has no positive (+) spikes between its rows of magnets. I would never sleep on any other magnetic mattress because of the potential long-term harmful effects from the positive spikes I have found in his competitors' products. I am so grateful that I now understand how and why this energy works.

Rotator Cuff

My oldest grandson threw a baseball to me one day, and I threw it back without a second thought. Something popped or tore in my right shoulder, and it was terribly painful. A year and a half later, it was still bothering me. This is another case where I never even thought to use a magnet. Later at a dinner with Dr. Bonlie and his wife, I told him about my shoulder. He looked at me in shock and said, "With all of the benefit you have had with the use of magnets, I can't believe you haven't used it on your shoulder." I realized that I must be a very slow learner. He was right—how could I have not thought of that until he pointed it out?

That night I slept with a magnet on my shoulder; there was a very noticeable improvement, and in 2 days, I was pain free once again. This had happened to me before. About a year before this incident, I had started using the magnets on my leg and knee when a doctor told me it was necessary to have a knee operation as the cartilage was torn. By sleeping with a 4 x 6 x 1 inch magnet, using the bio-north (negative) pole on my knee for about 3 months, I no longer needed an operation.

After so many successes, I now think of the magnets immediately when I have any accident or injury; they have never let me down.

Ruptured disk in My Neck

About a year and a half before I retired, I ruptured a disk in my neck. I went to many medical doctors, orthopedic specialists, and chiropractors, trying to find relief for the pain. I was pretty much nonfunctional for a long time and had been on glucosamine and chondroitin for some time. They helped, but I received only a 20 to 30 percent improvement. While at a health trade show, I ran into Dr. Bonlie, who could see I was in a lot of pain. He told me to start using the negative field of the ceramic magnet on my neck. He had given me this particular magnet about a year earlier for my prostate cancer.

It worked great, and within a few weeks I was totally pain free. For the first year or two, I relapsed from time to time, but as long as I had my magnet, I could control the pain in just a few minutes. It helps a great deal to have the right nutrients working with the magnetic energy for maximum healing potential. I had also been using a product called Pain Free at that time; it was a combination of glucosamine and chondroitin. It worked very well, but the FDA made them change their name. It is now called MoveFree. It is made by Schiff Corporation and is sold at Costco; it seems to work better than any other formula I have found.

Within less than a year of using the magnets and some stretching exercises, I had full range of motion without any pain. Nearly 20 years later, I still have full range of motion. At the first sign of a reoccurring pain, I use magnets a couple of times a year for just a few hours and remain pain free.

Knee

At the time of my retirement, I needed a knee operation. My right knee had been bothering me so badly that I didn't even want to drive around town. It seems funny that I never considered using my magnets for my knee after the previous success I had with my broken ribs, prostate, and the ruptured disk in my neck.

A doctor friend told me to take glucosamine and chondroitin to rebuild the cartilage, and the pain would go away. I did get relief from some of the supplements I took for my neck, back, and knee, but it seemed to quickly plateau after 3–4 months. I had been on the supplements for about 2 years and felt no further benefits to my knee. Just as with my rotator cuff, Dr. Bonlie reminded me at dinner to use my magnet. It worked.

I found, however, that after a few months, this also plateaued. Even though my knee was 90 percent better, it wasn't as good as new. I built a horseshoe device with the positive pole of one magnet on one side and opposed it with the negative pole of another. (They were both 4 x 6 x 1 inches.) I started using this while sleeping and I woke up every 1–2 hours to rotate the positive and negative sides. I noticed additional improvement the first night; within a month, I felt it was as good as new.

A few years later, I noticed some of the discomfort coming back. I was staying with a close friend in Mexico who had a magnet bed that was very unusual. Copper coils surround it in the shape of a cylinder; you lie in the center of it. It is an electromagnetic device. He told me that its research and development cost was $250,000—so high that it never went into production. Just one night in that bed and I had a very noticeable improvement with my knee as well as a couple of other more minor benefits.

Back Pain

My last shift on the fire department was December 4, 1989. I ruptured a disc in my neck at a large fire about a year and a half before I officially retired. I was pretty much nonfunctional for several years and went to many medical doctors, orthopedic doctors, therapists, and chiropractors to find relief from the pain. They finally told me to learn to live with it and that there was nothing further they could do for me. They said an operation would only give me a 10 percent chance of improvement and a 70 percent chance of decline.

I had lost so much range of motion that I couldn't drive safely. I wanted to travel but carrying a four- to five-pound bag was very painful. Being in constant pain made it difficult even to dress myself

A friend, Dr. John Lamar, started me on glucosamine and chondroitin, which helped. I improved about 20–30 percent, enough to travel and go to health trade shows. While at one of these, I ran into Dr. Bonlie, who could easily see that I was in a lot of pain. He told me to use the negative field of the five-pound magnet he had given me earlier to use for my prostate cancer.

The magnet worked great. In a few weeks, I was totally pain free. It worked equally well on my lower back. I would have relapses over the next year or two if I stopped using the magnet regularly, but it would control the pain in a few minutes when I did apply it. If I used it regularly for a few weeks, I could then go a few weeks without it. This felt like a miracle.

Soon I was able to do a stretching exercise program, and regained most of my range of motion within a year and all of it within a few more years.

I had chronic back pain for many years that cost me a lot of lost time from work. Dr. Robert Young, a PhD microbiologist, did a live blood cell analysis on me. He was able to tell me very much of my life's health history—from my prostate cancer to my back pain and many other issues over a 20-year period. He told me to start taking two nutrients, zinc and colloidal manganese, for a few days every time I felt pain or a noticeable weakness in my back.

I have no idea whether this will work for everyone, but those nutrients and the energy from Dr. Bonlie's magnetic mattress (which I started using about the same time) provided relief from my back and neck pain. I have not had any further pain of that type since 1994.

Hearing

Along with all my other health issues, I had lost about half the hearing in my left ear and about 25 percent in my right ear. I went to several doctors specializing in ears. They all tested me and told me that I had nerve damage. Each said that nothing could be done except to prescribe a hearing aid.

Getting old and fat was bad enough, but losing my hearing was more than I could handle. This was about the time I found out about my prostate cancer; I figured that I wouldn't live much longer, so who cared if I couldn't hear.

I happened to go to a naturopathic doctor with a friend in 1983. He stuck his finger down my throat and massaged the button that opened up the eustachian tubes and allowed my ear to drain into my throat. I got a definite improvement in my hearing. He told me to get some helichrysum oil, an essential oil that reportedly helps nerves grow. At that time, a half ounce of the oil was $85, and I just could not afford to pay that much. I met Dr. Jessie Partridge in 1992 and took one of his classes on magnetic healing. He said to use helichrysum and to tape a small magnet over my ear drum. I put a couple of drops of the oil in my ear at bedtime and taped a small negative magnet to my ear every night for a couple of months, and I got very good results with it.

I have since asked Dr. Bonlie about this, and his recommendation is not to sleep with it; just use the magnet for 20 minutes at a time, wait a few hours, and do it again. He reminded me that the long-term use of the negative field has detrimental effects because you always get a return positive field around the edge of a single magnet—so use a single magnet for shorter periods.

I must be hearing better now, as it has been years since anyone has hollered at me to turn down the television.

Heart

After 3 heart attacks in January 2001, I was having frequent angina, heart and chest pains. Twice while driving home, I had chest pains about an hour away from help, which added to my concern. I opted to try a 4 x 6 x 1 inch magnet with the negative side to my back behind my heart. I held another with the positive side over my heart and felt immediate relief from this experimental treatment.

At my earliest opportunity, I called Dr. Bonlie in Canada to ask for his advice about my use of magnets for my heart in this situation. He assured me that I had done the right thing, as it would relax the heart muscle and increase the oxygen flow to the heart. He also advised me to consider taking an oral chelator called DMSA to help remove heavy metal toxicity and the plaque that had caused the blockages that led to my heart attacks. He also recommended that I consider sleeping on a super-strength magnetic sleep pad, which I did; the rest of the story you can find in my chapter about the heart.

Smashed Finger

I smashed a finger so hard one time that the finger nail and the injured ends of it turned black and blue almost instantly, and the blood squirted 6 inches from the ruptured underside of the fingertip. I put a very strong negative magnet on the bottom and taped it down and another to the topside, negative to negative. Within a few minutes of the injury, 90 percent of the pain was gone; and I went back to work.

Within 24 hours, all the black and blue was gone. At that time, I started rotating positive on one side and a negative on the other every 20–30 minutes. Within 3 days, the rupture to the bottom end of my finger, where the blood came squirting out, was totally healed. Even the tenderness was gone, and I never lost the finger nail.

Teeth

I had 3 teeth pulled at different times one year, all from deep-seated, long-term infections. I tried using magnets on the teeth before I had them pulled, and they were very effective in reducing the pain and the swelling, but by themselves did not get rid of the infection.

After each extraction, I immediately placed a small neodymium magnet on the outside of my cheek (about the size of a dime) right over the gum where the tooth had been removed. Normally, after the numbness from the local injection wears off in 2–3 hours, I start taking pain pills. If I applied the magnet right away, I needed no further pain pills after the shots wore off.

For one extraction I had to sit in the dentist chair for an hour and a half. The tooth was broken at least 10 times and was removed in pieces. The dentist finally gave up and told me I would have to go to a dental surgeon and that there was a 3-hour wait. I was quite nervous about this, as I was sure she had done a lot of damage to my jawbone as well as to my gums. I left and was gone just a couple of minutes before realizing the pain shot I had received 2 hours before would not last another 3 hours before getting in to see the oral surgeon. I drove back to the dentist to get some pain pills just in case, but she had already gone to lunch.

I put the most powerful magnet I had on the spot. I recall thinking that I was sure it would help, but I never imagined how well. To my amazement, I remained pain free. When the surgeon got me in his chair, the procedure took only 10 minutes. We were both amazed that I was able to control the pain with the magnets. He made it seem very simple and made a quick $200. It was definitely worth it after the previous experience.

My Dad's Quadruple Bypass

A couple of years after I started using magnets, my father went into the hospital for a quadruple bypass. The following morning I went in to see him. As most of you may know, he had what looked like a zipper down the center of his chest. Both sides were severely bruised with red, black, and blue discolored flesh. I went home and made an 8-inch strip of dime-sized neodymium magnets. They were all close together and were sandwiched between 2 pieces of high-expansion foam. At the hospital I taped them to the worst side of his chest and told the nurse not to let anyone remove them. I was expecting an argument, but she said, "I have heard of this, but have never seen it done before." She covered him and said, "The doctor has already made his rounds, so we're good until morning."

The next morning I returned to make sure no one had removed the magnets. I did not have any to replace them if they were gone. When the doctor arrived and opened the dressing, I told him what I had done. He was very impressed with the accelerated healing and that there was no sign of bruising on the side where I had placed the magnets. The other side looked as bad as it had the day before, so their benefit was very apparent.

The doctor seemed to be as excited as I was to see what seemed like a miracle, which is what he called it. He said, "This is amazing. Let's see what it will do on the other side." I moved it, and the next day there was a very respectable improvement in the bruising. The strip wasn't long enough to cover the whole area, so it was easy to see that the bruising in the original area was nearly completely healed in 3 days. It took about 10 days for the part of the incision that didn't get magnetic treatment to heal completely.

By the second day, all of the veins in my father's hands and arms had collapsed, and there were huge black and blue spots. They had to give him IVs in his legs and feet. I had learned from trial and error that if a magnet could be applied to a bruised area quickly, the black and blue would be gone overnight. Waiting 48 hours, however, would mean it would take 3 days to get the same results. The negative field of a magnet works far better than ice to slow down swelling and bruising. The quicker you can get it on the injury site, the better results you will get. I have also found that the stronger the magnetic field, the better the results will be.

With all the interest and enthusiasm the doctor had expressed at first, I was amazed that he never asked where he could get more information on the subject or purchase some magnets for future research. However, two of the nurses were very interested in more information. It indeed made a believer out of my dad. Several of the nurses and some of his friends who had had similar operations told him they had never seen anyone heal as fast as he had.

My Father's Dog Bite

A few months later, my father came by my house to show me where a dog had bitten him—not just any ordinary dog, but a junkyard dog—an 80-pound pit bull. He had several serious puncture wounds on his hand and arm. He said that it was very painful, and that he had seen a doctor right after the incident. They gave him injections and cleaned up the wounds, but they still looked very bad with bruising and torn flesh right into the muscle. It had been about 12 hours since the dog had attacked him the evening before. I put magnets on 2 or 3 of the worst wounds. Most of the pain was gone within a few minutes. The next day, the injured areas with the magnets looked like they were week-old wounds with no bruising at all, but the one I did not put a magnet on was still quite bruised and had been the least severe of the 3 the day before.

My Yoga Injury

I had been going to a yoga class with my daughter, Laurie, for a couple of weeks, when I realized on April 15, 2010 that my right leg was not limbering up (although my left leg had been improving). I had broken my right ankle over 20 years before, and my right leg had remained stiffer than my left since then. I hadn't fully realized this until I started doing yoga. Trying to sit in a lotus position was very difficult, as my right leg would not relax enough to go past my right shoulder. At the time, I was not aware that yoga was unlike other exercise where the motto is "no pain, no gain." Instead, yoga is about listening to your body and easing off or stopping if anything hurts or overstretches it.

After a few weeks of class, I became very determined to force my right knee further to the right. One morning, I spent most of the class just working on this while everyone else did as the instructor suggested. By the end of the class, I could hardly get off the floor, I was in so much pain. I had damaged a tendon and/or ligament in my right hip and knee. I didn't realize until a week later how badly I had hurt myself. I kept trying to stretch it more and more, but very gently after that first morning.

I was still in a lot of pain 2 weeks after the incident. I realized then that it must be like a sprained ankle; it just wasn't getting better. Often, a badly sprained ankle takes several weeks or even 2–3 months to heal. I recall hearing many times that sometimes a sprain can be harder to heal than a break.

I still wasn't able to sleep on my right side, and it caused my right knee to ache as well. After living in a lot of pain for much of my life and then overcoming it some years earlier, this brought back some very unpleasant memories.

After this hip injury, I bought another one of Dr. Bonlie's magnetic mattress pads that goes with a single size bed. It is double thick for maximum gauss strength. I placed my 2 magnet pads under a 4-inch-thick mattress instead of under my regular mattress, which is approximately 12 inches thick. This provided a lot more gauss strength (gauss is a unit of measurement); and within 2 days, I was sleeping on my right side once again. Within 4 days, the pain in my right hip and knee was gone altogether.

Eye Story

I have a friend in Costa Rica who is a naturopathic doctor and an herbalist trained in Europe. His son has a degenerative eye disease. My friend has taken him to Cuba for treatment several times, and magnetic therapy is a large part of their program. He was very impressed with the results.

Below I have some more points of interest that you may want to read about:

Did you know that cockroaches and other insects get 90 percent of their energy from the earth's magnetic field, and that they do not have an immune system? They are very resistant to infectious diseases, and they do not get cancer. It kind of makes me wonder where we would be if all the billions of dollars spent on cancer research had gone instead to the study of cockroaches. I am pretty sure none of it has been spent on magnetic research or ozone. It's hard to believe that in most other countries, doctors can legally use both therapies and report getting great results but in the United States, most states won't allow doctors the discretion to do what they feel is in the best interest of their patients.

I have heard many success stories from people I have met at health expos. Only a few are even aware of the many benefits of magnets. This amazes me, and I think it is largely because multi-level marketing companies sell magnets but do not educate people about how and why they work so well. They just say to try it for a few days and that we'll see for ourselves. They do work well for a week or two; then all of our body's reserve energy is depleted and they no longer work. In fact, long-term use of bipolar magnets becomes very detrimental to our overall health.

Working with the earth's natural magnetic field, magnets have performed miracles in my life with accelerated healing and pain reduction. For thousands, if not millions (if we include the whole world I am sure), magnetic energy has worked very well. Many third world countries cannot afford high-priced modern medicine, so they are forced to stick with the old proven methods of treating themselves with magnets, diet, herbs, and home remedies. They just stick with what works. For a better understanding of why magnets are not a part of mainstream medicine in the United States, read the book *Suppressed Science*: "there is no money in it."

There is so much to learn about the use of magnets and so many benefits. I suggest that you order a book or two on the subject, if you are interested in doing your own research.

Who needs a magnetic mattress with a pure negative field? Everyone! This is the easiest way to start learning about the many benefits of magnetic energy, as there is no better way to learn than by experiencing it for ourselves.

Your education makes *Your Health Your Choice*. A few side notes you may find of interest:

The Healing Magnets: "It's not the pain relief alone that has doctors excited. Bio-magnetic therapy may be reversing the degeneration of joints and promoting the growth of new cartilage."

–Dr. Bob Arnot, MD, "Stop the Pain," *CBS This Morning*, February 9, 1993

This is only one of the many positive ways that magnets may improve our lives. Isn't it about time to get the facts?

I am positive the above is true from my own experience and the benefits I have received. Even if you have no need at this time, knowing what is available will be very valuable to you or a loved one at some time in the future.

"Humanity's common bond is that we either have a health issue or we will soon have one, even if it is just a common cold!"

There is no doubt about it: just like death and taxes, no one can avoid them and no one can avoid sickness, not even I. The difference between me and most others is that I have diligently documented my conditions and what I did to reverse them. With each one of my experiences, through prayer, someone came into my life to guide me to the answers I was seeking at the time. I am not smart enough to have figured any of this out myself, but I am open to receive all of God's blessings and appreciate those who are guided to take the time to teach me what I have learned in making my health my choice. I have complete confidence that this will continue for the rest of my life. Even though I expect to live beyond 150 years, the length of my life is not nearly as important to me as its quality. I love feeling 20 years old, and I expect that feeling to continue for many years to come.

Health is simple, as is anything you understand, and when you pray with the expectation of receiving what you want and need, you will receive it. The power of our minds is revealed in the Bible in many places, but most profound to me is Christ's statement, "The least among you can do all that I have done and even greater things."

I believe this power is in our minds; all of us have this ability. It is up to us to learn to use it—not just for our personal benefit, but for the benefit of humanity, as we are one with each other and one with God.

Live in love and light, as darkness cannot exist in the light of truth. When we can achieve this, Satan has no place left to live; he dwells in darkness where fear reigns, driven by negative energy.

I now enjoy every minute of every day, knowing that my energy, created by my positive mental attitude, fills my body, mind, and soul with light. Light is knowledge--- knowledge that leaves no room for negative energy and no room for Satan to exist.

After reviewing Dennis's information in the magnet therapy chapter, I endorse his enthusiastic stories of the use of magnet energy to accelerate healing. However, I would encourage everyone to consider the use of the Magnetico pad because there is absolutely no potential downside to sleeping on it. Using individual magnets requires a lot more understanding and education about using magnetic energy than Dennis has been able to put into a single chapter.

–Dr. Dean Bonlie

CHAPTER 5

Chronic Back and Neck Pain

I had a ruptured disk in my neck and several degenerative lower back disks that caused pain for many years, and I am now pain free with full range of motion.

In my first month on the fire department in 1961, I responded to a fire at an auto wrecking yard after dark. The department was so poorly funded and undermanned that we only had two men on our engine company. This was the norm, not the exception. I was the rookie, so I had to drive the truck and provide support to my lieutenant, Larry Sullivan.

He yelled over the sound of the engine for me to get a short pike pole from the top of the truck. The engine was revved up quite high and we were pumping 105 pounds of nozzle pressure. I quickly climbed to the top of the truck, grabbed the pole, and jumped off to get it to him as fast as possible. It was dark and difficult to see anything. Something caught my feet as I came down, and I twisted, landing on my right side.

Though it was very painful, my adrenalin was pumping; I got up and finished the job. We returned to the fire station, and I was able to get some sleep. But by the following morning, I could hardly get out of bed. My back injury was so severe that I couldn't work for several shifts. This was the beginning of my back problems, which lasted my entire career on the fire department.

Nearly every year, I would reinjure my back doing something—often this was simply bending over to pick something up, and often while at work. This gave me a bad reputation for abusing my sick leave, which I understood. If not for this ongoing back injury, I don't think I would have used a fourth of the sick leave that I did.

I feel it is very important to mention that in 1962, I had a back problem so severe that I couldn't get out of bed to go to a doctor. After a couple of days, my dad brought a friend over to examine me. Dr. Wade Sole, DC (doctor of chiropractic) told me that he could not find anything wrong with my back. He then asked for a urine sample in a clean glass. He held it to the light and showed me all the cloudy, stringy stuff in it. He said, "You just have a kidney infection," and prescribed a teaspoon of cumin, a simple spice I had in my spice rack, which was dissolved in warm water and drunk like a tea several times a day. I also had to drink several glasses a day of water with fresh-squeezed lemon, and also cranberry and cherry juice; he said that the pain would go away in a couple of days. He said I should continue for another couple of days afterward to make sure I didn't have a reoccurrence.

He was right on target. Then he told me to cut back on drinking Coke and Pepsi, which I had been drinking a 6-pack or more of per day. He lectured me for seemingly an hour about all the harmful effects they have on our bodies. At that age, it went in one ear and out the other; and I soon started back on the soft drinks after the pain was gone. I shortly thereafter had another reoccurrence; and once again, I was sure it was my back, but it turned out to be another kidney infection.

I must be a very slow learner, as I repeated this scenario several times over the next few years. The light finally came on after 8 or 10 times. I quit drinking soft drinks and have never had a kidney infection again.

I wanted to point this out for two reasons:

1. feel sure that some readers may find that what they believe to be back problems may just be kidney infections that can be addressed naturally, without antibiotics. Now that I understand the benefits of Sodium Chlorite (MMS) and Molecular Silver, both of which work far better than any antibiotic I have had occasion to use, I would definitely choose one or both to address any form of infection.

2. Soft drinks of all types are harmful to our health for many reasons.

Water, fresh fruit juice, and vegetable juice are all that I drink now. I do cheat a little, maybe once every month or two, and have a milkshake or something along those lines. While I was reversing my health issues, I was a puritan for several years. But now that I am feeling 20 years old, I feel comfortable indulging myself from time to time.

Nearly 20 years later, unless I do something to reinjure my neck or lower back, I no longer need to use the magnet in those areas. When that happens, it is only necessary to use the magnet a few times for 20–30 minutes; the injury heals quickly and permanently. And today I can pick up small refrigerators, heavy furniture, even bales of hay, and move them with no pain or fear of injury.

Most recently I got up at 4:00 a.m. on a Saturday morning, caught a plane to Spokane, Washington, and spent the day loading about 5 tons of products in a truck, along with taking care of other business; at 5:00 p.m. I was on the road. I drove 20 hours nonstop back to Las Vegas. I did take a little nap as dawn was approaching. I pulled off the road and slept 3 hours in the front seat of the truck. Arriving around 1:00 p.m. Sunday afternoon, I had lunch, rested for an hour, then unloaded the truck, finished by 8:00 p.m. that night. Being definitely tired, I quickly fell asleep, but was wide awake at 4:00 a.m. the next morning with only a few minor aches and pains. Again, this story illustrates why my physical condition continues to surprise me at 70 years of age.

In 1993 or so, I was at a health trade show in San Francisco and had the opportunity to hear a lecture by Dr. Robert Young, PhD in microbiology. He and his wife Shelley Young founded the Innerlight, pH Miracle, and Young pHorever companies. I was so impressed with what he said. Wrapping up his talk, he said he would be returning to his booth to perform a live blood cell analysis demonstration on someone from the audience in order to illustrate this point from his lecture.

I immediately moved to the back of the room; I was the first person at his booth and got my name at the top of the volunteer list. Most of the attendees were doctors in varying fields of health, and approximately 50 of them followed him back to his booth to watch.

I was astonished. While examining my blood sample, he said, "This part of the blood tells me that he had a lower back problem for approximately 20 years, this part tells me that he has been relatively pain free for the past few years, and this section tells me that the pain is coming back." He was absolutely right on his timeline and my health issues. Recently I had been feeling a weakness in my back, and even though the pain had not returned, I had become concerned about my back problem starting to plague me all over again. I couldn't imagine what gave him this extraordinary ability to see all of this in my blood.

He went on to say, "This area of the blood tells me that he has prostate cancer; although in its early stages, there is no question that it exists." Again I was shocked that he could see this, especially since the three urologists that I had seen over the last 3 or 4 years had told me that I had a lump that could be cancerous. Since they had no tests to tell for sure without doing a biopsy, I was reluctant to have one. I was concerned that once the cancer was opened up that it could spread.

I was fortunate enough to take Dr. Young to dinner that night. I spent about 3 hours one-on-one with him. I was anxious to get his opinion on what I could do about the prostate cancer and making sure the back problem did not reoccur. Again he surprised me when he said that my back problem, which had plagued me much of my life, was due to a lack of magnesium and zinc. He told me to pick up colloidal solutions of each at his booth the next day. I took 4 or 5 drops of each every morning and night until the weakness in my back went away.

He said that I would probably need to use these supplements once or twice a year as needed. Whenever the weakness began to come back, I would simply follow this regimen for a few days and it would go away. Once again, he was right on. Those first 2-ounce bottles I bought lasted 17 years. By following his advice, I have had no further back pain or feeling of weakness that lasted more than a few days.

For a quick synopsis of what benefited me: Initially I didn't have magnets, just the glucosamine and chondroitin. Once I added the magnets, I received a tremendous boost in benefits for my back, neck, and knee (please see Chapter 4 on magnetic healing for more in-depth information). A couple of years later, I added the magnesium and zinc to this protocol, which provided more benefit to my neck and back.

From a purely anecdotal perspective, I think that I got this incredible healing benefit from glucosamine and chondroitin, which I continued to take; they provided the cellular nutrients. Then the magnets provided the energy: the combination allowed everything to work synergistically. I had made little to no progress despite the thousands and thousands of dollars that State of Nevada Industrial Insurance spent on my rehabilitation using modern allopathic methods in the three previous years. This experience was a real eye opener about the benefit of alternative health practices. It really encouraged me to continue seeking alternative methods for all of my health issues.

Magnets have helped accelerate the healing of so many of my issues. It is unbelievable that this knowledge is not taught in United States schools. In Japan, you can buy magnets in drugstores.

I have been sleeping on Dr. Dean Bonlie's magnetic mattresses for nearly 20 years now, and it is great to wake up every morning feeling 100 percent pain free.

Remember, *Your Health is Your Choice*, as is your life. A positive mental attitude and determination to do whatever it takes to get the job done, in life and in health, allow us to achieve our desires.

CHAPTER 6

Prostate Cancer

In 1992, I started documenting my health issues and what I was doing to overcome them. In 1993, I wrote, "I cured myself of prostate cancer in 3 months." That is how I felt at the time, when I was just learning about health. Nearly 20 years later, I realize that we always carry cancer cells in our bodies, so I have come to accept the FDA stand that we should not use the word "cure." "Control" is probably the better choice of words, but it is still simple. If we create an internal environment that pathogens cannot tolerate, our body's own immune system is much more efficient and effective in healing itself, no matter what our symptoms or our diagnoses are.

I now believe that diseases are just symptoms of an imbalance in our internal environment that can be simply and inexpensively addressed in most cases.

Prostate Cancer and Prostatitis

The chronic prostatitis that became cancer plagued me for over 10 years. Three different urologists had me on antibiotics for months at a time. Prior to 1991, I still felt that if a medical doctor could not fix the problem, it couldn't be fixed; I couldn't imagine that I would be capable of learning anything my doctors didn't already know.

I first started noticing the symptoms, such as the increased frequency of urination, around 1983. It continued to get worse over the next few years very gradually, and knowing little about health then, I wasn't concerned much about it. Being over 40 and working with the fire department, my annual physical required me to have a prostate exam. It never entered my mind that I could have prostate cancer, and the doctors did not identify it.

In 1988, while working at Station 11, I had a conversation with Ron Drake, a close friend who had been in the first class of paramedics licensed by the State of Nevada many years earlier. He was the first person to tell me that I should have the doctors do a better job checking my prostate. Over the past year, he had noticed me getting up every hour or two at night to use the bathroom. He said, "There are other things that could cause that, but the prostate is the most likely."

When I retired in 1991, with the pain from my neck injury, my prostate problem, needing a knee operation, and having had to sit up to sleep for 3 years due to heartburn so bad I couldn't lie down, I was in misery most of the time. That was not a life. I felt that I was dying and that the doctors were doing more to kill me than cure me by keeping me on antibiotics. It took me a long time to realize that their treatment was like putting a Band-Aid on my problems or giving me an aspirin; it didn't address the underlying cause of anything, it just temporarily reduced the symptoms.

When I got up every hour or two to urinate, urine continued to drip and run down my leg for 2–3 minutes afterward. Each time this happened, I would recall a time in childhood at age 3, 4, or maybe 5, when I would eat watermelon before bed, then dream about urinating and wet the bed. I had changed the diapers of older relatives and became concerned that I might find myself in the same position. This was not a pleasant thought, but it motivated me to keep searching for something that would reverse this prospect.

My PSA test (the blood test for prostate cancer markers) was 77. A normal reading is under 4.0, but 1 is where it should be. Two different doctors diagnosed me with prostate cancer.

For a couple of years, I had tried every home remedy and herbal remedy I ran across for my prostatitis problem. After being diagnosed with cancer, I started getting very serious about finding a way to address it. When my dad and my uncle were my age, they had to have their prostates removed due to cancer. Both men totally lost their sex lives after the operation. I also had lost my physical desire without some form of stimulant by this time, and I hadn't had an operation.

A couple of years after my father's operation, he had a serious heart attack, and I rushed to the hospital to see him. He was in tremendous pain and was rubbing his left shoulder and sweating profusely. I asked him how he was doing, and he replied, "Not worth a damn!" I asked if he was in a lot of pain, and he replied, "Of course I am, but that isn't the problem." He said some worthless doctor had just told him it looked like he was going to have to give up half of his sex life. He said he asked the doctor, "Which half do you want me to give up, the talking about it or the thinking about it?"

This helped me to realize that keeping a sense of humor helps both the patient and the family. As I looked back on my father's joke while he was in such pain, I realized the positive effect it had on both of us. I decided right then never to complain but just to refuse to have a bad day or to let anyone upset me and ruin my day. I believe life should be about having fun and enjoying all it has to offer. All of life's challenges are just another learning opportunity, and that is why we are all here on earth anyway: to allow us to evolve spiritually.

By 1992, I had been diagnosed with prostate cancer, as stated in chapter 4 and I slept in an ozone bag every night as well. Explained in chapter 3, I can't say for sure what percentage of the role the magnets and the ozone played in overcoming the cancer, but the combination worked very well for me.

It wasn't until around 2006 that I noticed I was getting up once or twice a night to use the bathroom once again. I met Jim Humble around the first of February 2007, and he started me using Sodium Chlorite (MMS). I noticed several benefits. Getting up in the middle of the night decreased so gradually, I didn't even realize it was happening.

I used Sodium Chlorite (MMS) for 3 months straight. Then I went off for 3 months, then back on for 3. (I explain the regimen more completely in Chapter 21). I stopped using Sodium Chlorite (MMS) in the first week of 2008—not because it didn't work, but because I felt I didn't need it any longer. About a year later, I again got up once a night now and then, and by 2010, it was usually twice.

It has been slowly getting worse over the past couple of years, but not to the point of much concern. In fact, it only came to mind when I would wake up in the middle of the night needing to go to the bathroom. Consequently, I rarely thought to use a magnet throughout the day as I had in the past; as it was not nearly the major problem I had years before. It just didn't enter my mind.

The benefits of Photon Genie and Genius

After experiencing the Photon Genie and Genius at the Anti-Aging Show in Las Vegas (December 9 to 11, 2010), I was very impressed with the information about it. I listened to many doctors and health care practitioners there who had been using it with great success.

For the past 3-1/2 years, I have been putting in 16–20 hours of work a day and living on 3–4 hours of sleep a night. It is hard to keep the immune system working optimally without adequate sleep. I feel so good and am filled with such excitement about the reversal of all of my past health issues that it is hard for me to sleep. I wake up very early most mornings, feeling like jogging around the block and consumed with the desire to share this with everyone I meet.

(I often start the morning by writing down my thoughts about what I have done to feel so good. I don't want to forget anything, as I am usually doing several different things at once, and it is hard to evaluate whether it is just one or two things or a combination of several things that make the difference. Without writing these notes immediately, I forget the little things that have contributed to my feeling so young and vibrant once again.)

With my frequently inadequate sleep, I sometimes get the symptoms of a cold or sinus problem that move into my ears or throat. At times it causes me to wake up with tonsillitis 3 or 4 times every winter (I still have my tonsils). My use of oxidative therapies in the past 4 years has reduced these problems so that they don't last more than a few hours. This is very exciting in itself for me, and I cover it elsewhere in the book.

On December 11, 2010, the last day of the Anti-Aging Show:

I wrote the following (as I didn't want to forget this important information): I experienced the symptoms of the onset of a cold as for several nights in a row I have not had more than 3–4 hours' sleep per night. Shortly after walking into the trade show on the first day, Thursday morning, December 9, 2010, my nose plugged up and my ears filled up. There was no doubt in my mind that by nightfall I would have a full-blown cold and a sinus infection.

I was at the booth that displayed the Photon Genie when this occurred, so I used the unit around my sinuses, ears, and throat for about 15 minutes. My sinuses cleared up and my ears unplugged. I used the frequency probes for 15 more minutes; all signs of a cold and sinus issue disappeared and did not return.

When I ran across the Genie, it really wasn't within my budget; and because of its potential I felt it had, I asked for guidance. (I have studied a kinesiology, DVD course by Dr. Stephen and Beth Daniel of Quantum Techniques, in the use of muscle testing). When I asked if I should buy this device, the response was always an enthusiastic yes. I am so thankful I did; so far it has exceeded my expectations.

I will do my best to explain what this machine is and can do. A frequency generator in a large briefcase-sized unit is attached to 2 light probes, each about 1 foot long. 2 cigarette pack-sized boxes are wired to the generator. The 4 units all emit frequencies that create an inhospitable environment that pathogens cannot tolerate. When the 2 light probes and the 2 boxes are properly placed on the body, the energy frequencies pass through it just as the earth's magnetic energy does. These frequencies are critical to health and life; they add beneficial energy that helps the immune system to function better.

During the conference, I learned a great deal about the technology and received a lot of exposure to the energy frequencies the machines emitted. The next few days I slept 8 hours straight through the night without getting up once to use the bathroom. This effect lasted for nearly a week. I did not even feel the urge to jump out of bed and run to the bathroom first thing in the morning.

My prostate, bladder, and kidneys have not been working as they should for the past couple of years. I once again get up once or twice a night. My urine stream has also weakened noticeably. The incontinence has not returned nearly as badly as before, but my ability to hold it for long periods is greatly reduced. Now when I feel the urge to go, I can usually hold it for 30–45 minutes; but sometimes only for 10–15.

The 7th night I woke up once to go to the bathroom and I only got 5 hours sleep, so I caught a plane to Phoenix and bought a Photon Genie. The first night I used it, I slept 8 hours straight through. However, I was uncomfortable and had a very restless night, because I was using all 4 parts between my legs. I normally roll from side to side and am rarely even aware that I do this, as most of the time it doesn't wake me up enough for me to notice. When you have 2 hard plastic electrical devices about the size of a pack of cigarettes as well as 2 foot-long glass tubes in your crotch, all held in place with your shorts, it takes a little getting used to. The tubes light up 30 times per minute for 1 second each time and then go off for 1 second. When they light up, you hear it, and if the intensity is turned up too high, you get a little shock. It is not painful, but in your very tender and sensitive private parts, it can get your attention when you're trying to sleep.

I am sure you can see how uncomfortable all 4 of the devices in your shorts could be. It took me a few nights to get used to the idea, as I did have some concern that I would break the tubes and castrate myself in my sleep. The visual of that kept flashing through my mind during the initial few nights. At first, I only used them 2–3 hours a night, then I would take them out and sleep on through the night. By the end of the first week, I was able to sleep through the night without waking up or needing to go to the bathroom.

Even though I overcame prostate cancer and have had no symptoms for many years, recently some symptoms have gradually come back. These are the frequency of urination and loss of physical sexual desire. It has been over 20 years since I woke up with an erection without taking a stimulant.

After just 10 days sleeping with the Photon Genie, I woke up with an erection 2 mornings in a row. The fact that it's happening is very exciting to me (not that I necessarily care; what am I going to do with it?). It is difficult to evaluate the effects of nutrients and/or the benefits of any device. As I continue to learn more, I believe the return of sexual desire is a very positive sign that I am reversing my aging process even more.

I have found a product called Prostate Renew that is a combination of 10 herbs that synergistically work together to rebuild the prostate. It has the side benefit of acting as a precursor, allowing the body to produce testosterone naturally. Every night that I take one of these, I wake up with a smile on my face, as there is no doubt I am feeling much younger.

As of January 1, 2011, the benefits that I had seen in less than 2 weeks are the following improvements:

A. Improved sleeping

B. Reduction in dribbling or dreams of urinating in my sleep

C. A minor strengthening of my urinary stream

D. Improvement in sexual desire

Possible downsides to my experience:

A. I gained 10 pounds in the same 2 weeks. It was too early to tell if there was a relationship to the use of the Photon Genie as of January 1. I usually gain a few pounds over the Christmas holidays, but 10 is more than usual. I would observe whether it came off easily over the next week or not. When one feels 20 years old, metabolism is very good; I normally don't need to be concerned about a 5–10-pound fluctuation.

B. The time it takes to get used to sleeping with the devices. If you can sleep on your back, it shouldn't be a problem; but if you roll from side to side as I do, it may take a while to get comfortable. I suggest that if you buy or lease a device, keep trying even for an hour or two and eventually you may be able to sleep through the night.

Waking on January 1, I was so focused on writing this story that I didn't even realize that I had a head cold developing until I could no longer breathe out of either nostril. New Year's Eve was very cold in Las Vegas; the wind through my bedroom window was blowing directly on my face and kept my room temperature at approximately 65 °F to 68 °F.

I took the probes from my crotch area, wiped them off with baby wipes, and placed them alternately at each side of my nose and into my nostrils. Within 5 minutes, I was able to blow my nose; and within ten, I could breathe normally through my left nostril. It took about an hour for both of them to clear up, but I kept the probes in place for another hour just to make sure the cold didn't come back. I have written more information on the Photon Genie in chapter 19. I have found many beneficial uses for it over the past year.

January 14, 2011, I had lost the weight I had gained without trying to diet. I did it by just maintaining my normal routine and not having snacks around to tempt me.

Still lying in bed, contemplating all that I have learned about health over the past 20 years, I recalled one of my proudest moments at an anti-aging health show in 2003. Dr. Wang, who was working with an enzyme company, had been good enough to spend over an hour with me, explaining the many benefits of enzymes and how they can eat scar tissue as well as their value in all cellular repair.

At lunch about a half hour later, I was speaking with a doctor beside me when a Chinese doctor from Canada sat at our table. He was one of the guest speakers at this convention, and had an entourage of about 10 other medical doctors who filled in the rest of the seats at the table. A few more just stood around listening.

Everyone was quiet except the doctor beside me and myself, who were still conversing about how simple health can be. We seemed to be on the same page about many points; furthermore, it was not often that a medical doctor was open to engage in a conversation with me, a layman. The doctor said something I agreed with, and I said, "I am sure you are right. I expect to still be here 100 years from now, living a very active, healthy, productive, and fun-filled life."

The Chinese doctor sitting across from me loudly butted into our conversation, making sure everyone heard him. He said to me, "That is the stupidest statement I have ever heard. What kind of doctor are you anyway?" Everyone around the table wanted to hear more.

I replied, "I am not a doctor; I was a fireman for 30 years and felt 90 years old when I retired 12 years ago, and I feel 30 years old today. Now, 8 years later, I feel like I am 20. I have successfully overcome prostate cancer. I have also cleared the blockages that caused 3 heart attacks and repaired the heart damage from them with magnet therapy. Now that I understand oxidative therapies, I don't believe there is a disease that can harm me."

He responded, "Well, that is still a stupid statement. You can't heal a damaged kidney. What would you do about that?" I replied humbly, "I have no idea, as I have never had that problem, but I have no doubt that, through prayer, someone would come into my life who would help me find the answer." Even though he was very dominating and disrespectful in his approach, I never took offense to what he said. Remaining eager to learn all I could about health, I welcomed everyone's input, and he was obviously a very knowledgeable man.

I guess he was embarrassed that he didn't back me down and that I didn't just quietly leave the table. Still, he tried 3 more times to push me into to saying something he could dispute to make me look like I didn't have any business sitting at the same table with him. The third time, he asked, "Where would you even start to reverse kidney damage?" I replied, "I would probably start by looking into enzyme therapy." I just learned about it from Dr. Wang, who taught me that enzymes are necessary for all cellular repair and can eat scar tissue."

The doctor cocked his head, looked up in the air without a word, reached into his pocket, pulled out his business card, and started writing on it. He wrote his personal cell phone number and e-mail address and handed the card to me, saying, "I want to keep track of you."

By now we had all finished lunch and started to walk away. Three of the doctors present came to me at once and asked, "Did he really give you his cell phone number?" I said, "I haven't tried to call him, so I can't say for sure, but you all heard what he said." One doctor said, "I have worked with him for 3 years now, and I don't even have his cell number."

It was very exciting to receive that type of feedback from a doctor of his stature. I went immediately back to Dr. Wang. He was kind enough to spend a few extra hours with me, explaining more about enzymes, their benefit, and how and why they work.

I can't say for sure what is making the difference in my kidneys, bladder, and prostate, as I have only this story to tell. Nevertheless, I hope to better my understanding of what combination of things can work together to heal these organs. I think that the minerals I use (which I believe are the best in the world) are basic requirements for enzymes to build the foundation of cellular health.

ASEA (explained further in chapter 7) assists cellular communication and the amino acid that provides nutrition. The Genie and Dr. Bonlie's magnetic mattress provide the energy to heal these vital organs. This makes perfect sense to me now, understanding the interrelationship between energy, these nutrients, and cellular health.

Health Made Simple

Since I feel 20 years old now, I don't want to be plagued with the many symptoms of disease or old age. As I have said, I believe that all health issues are just signs of imbalance in the body's internal environment. Everyone promotes antioxidants, yet they do not realize that oxidants are every bit as important, if not more so. If we maintain a proper balance of friendly digestive flora, we will seldom have a sickness or disease. Furthermore, if we learn to cleanse, detox, rid our bodies of pathogens, and reduce our viral load and environmental toxins, our bodies can heal themselves more efficiently.

Never forget Deepak Chopra's advice: "We need 6 or 7 hours of sleep a night. One thing that can help us to relax and center the mind is to close the right nostril and breathe in through the left, then reverse: close the left nostril and breathe out with the right." He explained this technique on the *Dr. Oz* television show on January 5, 2011; it works very well for me. Dr. Mercola's January 8, 2011 newsletter was about sleep. Among other things, he said that using a computer or having a light on at night will keep us from getting the type of sleep necessary to maintain health, because they often produce insomnia.

We are energy beings, so understanding how to use different types of energy will soon enable us to manifest our own health needs, wants and desires, and our destinies. I have no doubt that energy is the future of medicine. As I learn more from the many people coming into my life, the future looks exciting. Dark forces cannot survive in the light. We will be a part of changing the world and making it a better place for all.

This is my prayer; and I manifest it every day through my, thoughts, actions, visualizations, and emotions.

Here is a simple formula that my friend Chik Shank taught me for manifesting needs, wants, and desires: "Thought + Emotion = It." "It" is whatever it is you desire. Christ said, *"The least among you can do all that I have done, and even greater things."* The Bible says, "With the faith of a mustard seed we can move a mountain."

Energy is not new; it is suppressed science, as Satan does not want us to know how powerful we are. Our minds, hearts, and souls are one with God, giving us limitless power over our physical abilities on earth. Living in love and light will open the doors to this knowledge as we all learn to manifest our needs, wants, and desires; this ability is within us.

CHAPTER 7

Eyes

After 25 years of bifocals, I no longer need glasses. When I got my pilot's license in 1970, I did not need glasses; however, by 1972, I did. My ophthalmologist told me that it's just a part of getting old. I said that I was just a kid in my early thirties and that this was unacceptable. I asked what else was available beside glasses. He had no other suggestions. I went to several other doctors over the years to stop the degeneration of my eyesight. Without exception, they all gave me the same answer, "What do you expect? You're getting older, and that is what happens." I didn't want to believe it, but when I couldn't find a doctor who could offer me any hope at all, what else could I do but accept this as the truth?

I did accept it until I started chelation treatments to improve my memory and increase my energy levels. By the time I had 7 or 8 treatments, I noticed improvement in my short-term memory, energy level, and unexpected improvement in my eyesight. I felt like walking and doing things that I didn't have the energy to do before the treatments.

There were usually several patients being treated at the same time. I found the knowledge the others had to offer to be as valuable as the treatment itself. One patient pointed out that chelation is primarily a form of cleansing the circulatory system, which the doctor confirmed. It occurred to me that if my memory and eyesight improved and my energy level increased from cleansing, I might be able to reverse other health problems with other types of cleansing and detoxing.

I started going to health trade shows, attending one or two a month wherever I could find them. They usually lasted 3 or 4 days and would include dozens of doctors and health care professionals speaking on different subjects each hour of every day. It became addictive, like going to a smorgasbord and eating until I was sick. I was usually torn between two or three different speakers who were lecturing at the same time. Sometimes I tried to cover two at once if they were next to each other or across the hall, running back and forth between them trying to catch the highlights. If I liked them both, which I frequently did, I would buy their books and tapes to take home with me.

In the first few years, I spent thousands of dollars on books, tapes, and courses from dozens of doctors and health care professionals. Soon I understood how a doctor could spend a couple hundred thousand dollars on education. Over the past 20 years, I have spent that much or more, including travel expenses. That's not counting what my insurance companies have paid for tests, procedures, X-rays, MRIs, and doctors' visits. (Fortunately, the fire department provided high-quality medical insurance, and I definitely took advantage of it.)

Though I found very little benefit from the allopathic approach to either diagnosing or treating my health issues, the medical test results have been helpful. They provided me with an idea of what to look for so my body can heal itself. It absolutely amazes me that I have met so few allopathic physicians who understand at all how simple health can be. They all seem to be so fixated on their specific field of expertise that they cannot see the forest for the trees. Many of them feel their own little piece of the puzzle gives them the whole picture of health.

I had lost a lot of respect for doctors who practiced conventional medicine by the time I met Dr. Debora Banker. After a 2-hour workshop on her eye exercises, I saw enough improvement to show that, with a little more work, I would never need glasses again. From the moment I walked out of the workshop, I never *did* put them on again. I still refer to her kit, which teaches how to do her program, and recommend it to others. Any time I notice a little deterioration in my eyesight, I just do more eye exercises and take the nutrients she recommends.

A combination of chelation, eye exercises, and nutrition worked for me, and over 10 years later, I did not need glasses. Now, 20 years later, I am still not wearing glasses, but since I could detect that my eyes were fading a little, I went to an ophthalmologist in Las Vegas on March 29, 2011. The exam indicated my vision was 20/30 with no eye health concerns. Although the doctor told me it could easily be corrected to 20/20, I really do not need to use glasses except in poor light with small print. I carry a small pair of dollar store cheaters in my wallet, but I have not used them once in over a year. It is imperative for me to resume eye exercises to see if I can get back to 20/20, since the biannual flight exam for my pilot's license is coming up and I will need to pass another eye exam to be current.

Our eyes are controlled by muscles that allow us to focus and bring images into our minds in a manner we can recognize. Like all muscles, they need to be exercised. "The human body is made up of some 400 muscles, evolved through centuries of physical activity. Unless these are used, they will deteriorate," says Dr. Eugene L. Fisk. Dr. Deborah Banker pointed out that glasses make our eyes lazy and weak and should be used as little as possible, while we should strengthen our eyes through nutrition and exercise. I found this to be true, but never heard her talk about the benefits of chelation. I believe the improvement in my eyesight was largely because I had chelation done first. It cleansed the circulatory system and increased blood supply, which set the stage for the benefits of eye exercises and added nutrition.

Dr. Banker designed her eye exercises specifically to improve circulation to and from the head and eye area. These exercises are somewhat like yoga stretches. She says that people of all ages have incorporated these powerful exercises into their lives; when I met her, she claimed that only once in her career did she have to resort to an operation to keep someone from needing glasses. The exercises take 15–20 minutes to complete and should be done 3–4 days a week, depending upon the individual's condition.

Constant multitasking has inspired my goal to achieve two years of experience in every year of my life. Soon I was doing the eye exercises while driving around town. At every stop light, I would focus on the car in front of me and exercise my eyes. Doing this a minute or two at a time, 20 or 30 times a day, worked very well for me.

About 15 years later, I woke up one morning and recognized another decline in my eyesight. It was such a subtle change that I had hardly noticed it. In March 2007, approximately 6 weeks after starting Sodium Chlorite (MMS), I woke up and realized I could see much better. I was staying with Jim Humble in Sonora, Mexico, and told him of my experience. The first thing he said was that Sodium Chlorite (MMS) could not chelate.

Over the following couple of months, we discussed it further and figured out that it was the oxidation of the plaque that allowed the increase in blood flow, allowing a similar benefit to chelation.

I did not accomplish this overnight. There was much trial and error and a lot of prayer. It takes time and commitment, 7 days a week, to succeed. My initial leap of faith in my ability to learn anything allowed me to make a difference in my own health. At retirement, I thought only a doctor could heal me. Once I began to see how simple health could be, my determination to succeed compensated for my lack of education in this field.

In 1991, I started on my quest for knowledge. Like many today, I figured if a doctor couldn't figure out how to fix my many health problems, it must be way beyond my ability to help myself.

I now know that only the body can heal itself, and I believe it doesn't matter whether it is our eyes, ears, or any other organs; only we can make a difference. It is imperative to provide the body with the nutrition and energy it needs to do the job of supporting the immune system. Maintaining the balance in internal environment, cleansing, detoxing, the right nutrition, and a little exercise allow us to heal ourselves of anything. Eye diseases, like all other ailments, require an aggressive and effective self-help therapy that we can learn, but it takes determination and dedication to follow the required protocols.

The nutrients I used are as follows:

1. Bilberry: It helps to remove toxins from the retina.

2. Eyebright: It helps strengthen the eyes.

3. Juniper berries: For optic nerve weakness.

4. Vitamin C.

5. Vitamin B complex: A very good and affordable source is baker's yeast—not the brewer's yeast that is normally used to ferment bread and alcohol, but nutritional baker's yeast that comes in a cake (not granulated). Be careful not to overdo this, as it supports fungal growth (as does fermented food); and if you have a health challenge that could be fungal related, it's best to not take any vitamin Bs until you have the fungus under control.

6. Minerals and trace minerals: A balance of all known beneficial minerals along with trace minerals that are in an angstrom size, allowing for 100 percent absorption at the cellular level. I feel certain that there are hundreds, if not thousands, of nanosize minerals that scientists have not discovered yet that benefit the body and are more likely to be in minerals derived from a whole food source.

   Colloids (like colloidal silver) and other complex minerals are all in particle size of approximately a micron. A human hair is about 50 microns wide. An angstrom is 10,000 times smaller than a micron. One unit of "angstrom" is 10 billion times smaller than a meter. That equals .5 million times smaller than a single hair. That is why it is 100 percent bioavailable at the cellular level. (*Size conversion from* http://www.unitconversion.org/unit_converter/length.html)

7. Zinc: Helps with tissue repair.

I also use a 2/3 magnesium to 1/3 calcium supplement—not for the eyes, but to help bones remain strong and pliable. This helps a great deal with cellular communication and heart health. It is also 100 percent bioavailable and is made by the same manufacturer that makes the other minerals I use, so I thought I would mention it here. There are many other foods and herbs that may help; the list above is just some of what I have taken, and they work for me. I do not take all of them all the time.

I will probably state this several times in my book, but I do believe one of the most important things I ever learned in my life is the proper way to use kinesiology to test everything I eat and do for my health. Kinesiology is the science of muscle movement and testing. I use a pendulum for that purpose. If you would like to learn more about this subject, you can go to www.drhealthclub.com for links. Also check out my friend Dr. Stephen Daniel's website, www.quantumtechques.com. He sells very inexpensive, easy-to-understand DVDs that explain this type of testing and teach many ways to do it. It can really change your life.

Now that I have finally learned how to use my pendulum, I muscle test nearly everything I put into my mouth, including supplements and every meal to test what I should eat. Muscle testing accesses the body's innate intelligence through the use of a pendulum. I wear mine around my neck 24 hours a day, 7 days

> a week. It also provides an energy block from harmful electromagnetic radiation (EMR). Most people purchase pendulums from a store that sells psychic energy devices; most are inexpensive quartz crystals. The one I prefer has added frequencies that give me more confidence in the information I get as well as more protection from harmful EMR. It is hard for me to imagine that I was skeptical about muscle testing for 20–30 years until I finally understood how it works, and I now believe it is the most accurate way to test anything related to health.

Since Dr. Deborah Banker passed away, I have been recommending the EYEPORT Vision Training System designed by Dr. Jacob Lieberman. Although I met Dr. Banker and used her course for my own eyes several years before I was aware of Dr. Lieberman, I had spoken with him many times. His knowledge, generosity, and patience in explaining things impressed me. I have referred many people to his website, and everyone has been pleased with the benefit they have received from his books and vision training system.

Dr. Lieberman is one of the increasing number of people I know who understand that energy plays a big part in our ability to heal ourselves. His website is www.exerciseyoureyes.com.

CHAPTER 8

Hearing Loss

I can hear again! I first noticed my hearing loss in the 1970s when I was tested in a fire department annual physical. Over a few years, three doctors assured me that my loss of hearing was due to nerve damage and that nothing could be done. They said that it was most likely due to the fire truck's siren. They told me that a hearing aid was imperative, or else my hearing would not only get worse, it would affect the other ear as well. My hearing did get worse: more and more people told me to TURN DOWN THE TV in a very loud, irritated voice, just as you see in a cartoon at the movies.

I felt the hearing loss could very well be due to a genetic weakness in my family, since my mother, uncle, and grandmother all had to wear hearing aids in their left ear as far back as I could remember. (My sister also had hearing loss in the same ear, but not to the extent of needing a hearing aid.) They have all had problems with their hearing aids not working, squealing, or not fitting correctly. When I explained this to the doctors, their advice was to put it off as long as possible and get a second opinion.

In the next several years, I went to other specialists hoping to find new technology. At the time, I had so many other health problems that I felt my hearing was the least of my health challenges. Getting old and fat was bad enough; losing my hearing was just one more inconvenience.

I will give you some ideas of what you may be able to do if you have hearing loss, since I have never used a hearing aid and am hearing fine at this time. My hearing is not perfect, but it has dramatically improved over what it was 20 years ago, with no help from any of the ear specialists I've seen.

Eustachian Tubes

I happened to go to a naturopathic doctor with a friend while on vacation in Hawaii around 1983 or 1984. I told him about my hearing problem and asked if he had any ideas. He said, "I don't know if this technique will help the problem, but I am sure it won't hurt to try. If you continue to do it yourself, you will definitely see an improvement."

He had me open my mouth, and he stuck his index finger in over the top back part of my tongue and down my throat. At the point where the index finger is down as far as it will go, there is a little button on each side of the throat that is a drain for your eustachian tubes. They are just behind and below where the tongue becomes the throat, just beyond the uvula. They allow the inner ear and sinus to drain. It is quite common for the tubes to get blocked from an infection or just debris backing up, stopping the natural drainage from the sinuses and ears.

When the eustachian tubes are blocked, it can feel like a minor to a major pressure buildup, depending on severity. My buildup had been very slow, over more than a ten-year period, and I never noticed the pressure until it was released. The first time the doctor showed me how to do this, I was sure I would throw up all over him. It is easier to do myself than it was to have him do it to me.

It helped a lot if I sat up with a garbage can in my lap, negating worry about the consequences of throwing up all over the room; fortunately, that never happened. I used my right hand to work the left side of my throat and the left for the right side. By using a self-hypnosis technique and completely relaxing myself mentally, I was able to avoid the gag reflex by my third attempt. The first 3 times, I put my finger down my throat 10–15 times for a second or two. It wasn't long before I could put it there and keep it there for 20–30 seconds, gently massaging the buttons on the inside of my throat. After a few hours, I would do it again, just once each time for 20–30 seconds on each side.

I did both sides in case there might be blockage that I wasn't aware of, and I kept hoping I might get a little improvement in my right ear as well. My right side always seemed normal, even though one of the doctors made me aware that I had some loss of hearing there also. I never got any improvement on the right side from this procedure, but I kept trying both sides every time.

Only occasionally would I feel a minor pressure release that would translate to a minor improvement in my hearing. That is what encouraged me to continue to do this procedure. Over the next few months, I did this many times and probably got a 30 to 40 percent hearing increase in my left ear; when it plateaued, I quit. The blockage has come back many times over the past 30 years, but I recognize it immediately and do this procedure again until it clears up. I can still put my finger all the way down my throat without triggering a gag reflex, so it was only difficult the first few times.

I explained to the doctor in Hawaii that several ear doctors had recently told me my hearing loss was from nerve damage and that there was nothing I could do about it except to wear a hearing aid. He said, "I feel the body can heal anything and everything when it has the opportunity to work with the proper nutrients." He suggested I get some helichrysum, an essential oil that reportedly helps nerves grow. He explained that if I put a couple of drops in my ear at bedtime, it would help regrow any damaged nerves. I did not follow his advice then, because the oil is extremely difficult to find and very expensive. However, I never forgot what he told me; just opening my eustachian tubes had made a huge difference in my ability to hear, giving me a great deal of confidence in his knowledge. I soon forgot the name of the oil, and it did not enter my mind again for nearly ten years until I once again had another doctor bring it back to my attention. In a lecture in 1994 I heard on essential oils, I ordered immediately; a half-ounce bottle that cost $85, which was difficult for me to afford, but I did it anyway and it did help.

Just a couple of added thoughts, alpha lipoic acid has high antioxidant properties and increases glutathione levels, which play a big role in dissolving toxic substances in the liver. Coffee enemas will also increase the natural production of glutathione as well (see more about this in Chapter 20). In addition, alpha lipoic acid reportedly helps regrow nerve damage as well, and I have had some benefit from using it on my feet. At the time I learned about this, around 2004, hearing was no longer a noticeable problem for me, so I have not tried to use it on my ears.

Ear Candling

In 1991, I met a woman in a health food store who recommended ear candling. An ear candle is approximately a foot-long, cotton linen cloth soaked in beeswax and rolled into a cone that resembles a long, hollow candle. She sold me a pair of candles for $10 and told me how to use them. You lie on one side while someone puts the cone in your ear and lights it with a match. It takes 10–12 minutes to burn down. The closer it gets to your ear, the hotter it naturally becomes and the more benefit it gives. The heat melts the wax in your ear and creates an updraft, sucking the wax, old infection, and other debris up into the candle or cone.

A friend and I followed her instructions exactly, and it worked very well. There was a big improvement in my hearing. I highly recommend that everyone try this. Several ear specialists did nothing for me, yet this simple, inexpensive treatment made a major difference.

You cannot do this by yourself; you must have a helper. If you cannot find someone to help you, it is worth paying someone with experience the first time or two. After you have seen it done a couple of times, you will probably feel confident enough to assist a friend or family member, and then he or she can reciprocate.

To protect the ear from falling sparks and embers, I perform the procedure in the following way:

- Cut a small hole in the center of a paper plate, just large enough to allow the small end of the candle to slip through before entering the ear. Put a slit in a paper towel, wet it, and put it over the plate. Then put the candle through both holes.

- Use a pair of very good scissors to cut the end of the candle as it burns down.

- Drop the embers into a small bowl of water that is close by, every couple of minutes. This eliminates the risk of the embers getting too long and dropping onto the ear, or getting into the hair of the person being treated.

- It is a good idea to have a spray bottle of water close by for added safety.

If you feel better about professional help, check to see if local chiropractors do this procedure. I have met several that do and have even taken a class in it from one. My mother and grandmother told me that when I was young, most medical doctors did this for their patients, but I guess they have all had to give it up due to the high cost of malpractice insurance. I doubt you could find a practicing medical doctor who currently performs it, or even remembers it being done.

The woman from the health food store told me to be sure to put hydrogen peroxide in my ear after every time to kill any remaining infection that might still be there. She used an eyedropper and put a few drops in each ear 2 or 3 times, as she said my ears were exceptionally dirty. I assumed that all the smoke I was exposed to as a fireman for 30 years might have contributed a great deal. Smoke can be irritating to sensitive tissue such as eyes and ears.

Even though I now knew what to do and how to do it, I still was not confident enough to candle myself. It was some time before I found someone who had done it before and was willing to assist me. At that time, I hadn't been into alternative health very long and didn't know many people who were. Now I know hundreds who are into treating themselves, and many have used ear candling successfully. With the rising cost of health care and the lack of permanent benefit that mainstream medicine offers, it is increasingly important to learn how to maintain optimum health yourself.

I added this therapy to all the other things I was doing, and my healing process has continued to improve. No one has asked me for several years now to turn down the television. I highly recommend these therapies to everyone who has hearing loss.

Magnets

In 1994 I finally ordered some helichrysum oil, but while I waited for it to arrive, I took another seminar on magnetic healing by Dr. Jesse Partridge. He claimed to have had good results with hearing problems. I spent more than $800 on all of his books and tapes plus an assortment of magnets. He recommended that I sleep with a small neodymium magnet taped over my ear with the negative side down. He also suggested taping them to my ears while bouncing on a mini trampoline (rebounding).

Once my helichrysum oil arrived, I used it with the magnets and noticed an improvement within a couple of weeks. Using the tip of my little finger, I rubbed a couple of drops on the inside of my ear as far down as I could reach. Now focused on my hearing, I recalled my experience in Hawaii and resumed my finger down the throat routine. For a couple of weeks, I did all of the above while rebounding in the evening before bed but gave up after 2 weeks, as I had no noticeable benefit from adding rebounding. I think I had already reached a plateau.

Knowing what I know now, I would not sleep with magnets taped to my ears; I would only use them while rebounding. It is not a good idea to use a powerful magnet on your head for over 20 minutes at a time. However, I believe that using magnets with helichrysum oil and alpha lipoic acid would be very helpful.

My hearing problem may not be the same as yours, but I was able to find options when doctors told me there were none. This story may encourage you to keep looking even beyond where I needed to go to regain my hearing.

Tinnitus

Following Dr. Bonlie's advice, I started using a mini trampoline along with all the other remedies to treat my tinnitus. At the time I did not know that that tinnitus can be addressed through diet alone. It is usually caused by a high-fat and high-sugar diet. Since fat and sugar were much of what I ate, adding the rebounder proved to be a waste of time. Since then, staying away from high-fat, high-sugar foods has worked well for me.

Although rebounding did not help with my tinnitus, I feel it is so important that I have devoted Chapter12 to providing more in-depth information on it.(A rebounder is a small trampoline that exercises every cell in the body simultaneously, including those in the ears and eyes.)

I believe all of the complementary modalities above helped me regain my hearing. Only the opening of the eustachian tubes and the ear candling gave me a fast, noticeable difference in my hearing; when the pressure was released on several occasions, it was noticeable right away. All the rest of these things were very subtle. I used the combination for probably close to a year, on and off, until I stopped after noticing no benefit for a long while. I may never get back to perfect hearing, but at least it has improved enough to change my life.

The more serious a problem is, the more we notice any improvement. When we plateau, we seldom notice a continual, subtle improvement. Most people, like me, will quit doing whatever was working when they plateau and are no longer seeing improvement daily, since they think the protocol no longer works.

I have plateaued to the point I was not noticing improvements many times. This does not mean there were no continued benefits; they were just too slow to be noticeable. Being very impatient, I like to see improvements yesterday, but daily is acceptable, or at least weekly. If I don't notice improvements at least weekly, I normally move on to something else. It is quite possible that many of the things I have tried would have worked to some degree if I had stuck with them longer, but my impatience gets the best of me quite often.

My last ear problem started in February of 2002, shortly after my heart attack. I had been using ozone 10–12 hours a night for a week, with the aforementioned leakage. I developed a bad cough that aggravated my sinuses. Afraid to continue using the ozone because of my lungs, I ended up with a gland and sinus infection.

I went to Southern California to see my youngest son and his family for a few days. While I was there, it was cold and damp; a sinus infection evolved into a cold. One morning I blew my nose and some mucus backed up into my eustachian tubes. I lost about 50 percent of my hearing in my right ear and 20 percent in my left ear in just the time it took to blow my nose. By that night, I had lost about 90 percent of the hearing in my right ear and 50 percent in my left ear as the infection rapidly set in.

I didn't have any of my books, notes, or equipment with me to try treating it myself. This was a terrible feeling; while I was thinking about writing my book, all these health problems continued to overwhelm me. The problems were bad enough in themselves, but to have them without anything I could help myself with threatened my dream of writing. I wondered what knowledge I could offer others when I couldn't even help myself with a simple ear infection. Today I know that Sodium Chlorite (MMS) and Molecula Silver most likely would have taken care of the infection within a few hours.

For Southern California, it was an unusually cold day in February; as night fell, the pressure on my eardrum intensified. I was in a lot of pain and decided to go to the emergency room at a nearby hospital. I was pleasantly surprised to find a group of caring people from the time I walked into admitting, right through to the ER doctor. They got me in and out in an hour and a half with prescriptions for antibiotics and pain pills. The pills nauseated me, but at least I was able to go to sleep. Shortly after waking, I started throwing up every 1–2 hours.

Finally, I went to a close-by Quick Care clinic. Once again, the staff and doctor were very friendly and helpful, and the visit took only an hour and a half. They gave me a shot of antibiotics and one for nausea, and antibiotic eardrops. Everything seemed to be working well; at least the pain was under control and the nausea was gone.

A week later, the hearing in my right ear was at a 90 percent loss and the loss in the left was 25 percent. Once back home, I was using the same modalities that I used to be successful with, but they were not working.

As I prayed about this, I felt assured that God would guide me down the right path to enlightenment and the right people would come into my life to help me find the right solutions.

Now that I understand Sodium Chlorite (MMS) and ozone, which oxidize pathogens, it is a simple matter. If I had gargled with ozonized warm salt water, the problem would have been gone in a few hours. For 5 years now I have used Sodium Chlorite (MMS) and Molecula Silver many times for tonsillitis and sore throats—for myself and some of my children and grandchildren. We always start at the first sign of a cold and it is gone within hours. In contrast, it has been my experience that a few days' delay in using Sodium Chlorite (MMS) or Molecula Silver will mean a few days to overcome a cold.

One new thing I learned with this last health issue that has helped me to drain the eustachian tube is the use of niacin (not timed-release niacin). A chiropractor friend suggested trying niacin to open up my ears. I would ingest 500 milligrams on an empty stomach (though starting at lower doses is highly recommended; e.g., 50 to 100 milligrams, then increase to tolerance), then wait about 30 to 40 minutes, and it really lights me up. It causes flushing and tingling in my face and neck, and I can feel it opening up my ears. Sometimes they will start popping just like when driving up and down a mountain. I find putting my finger down my throat during the flush gets much better results.

Taking the niacin on an empty stomach works best, but if you do not feel the necessary flush, drink a glass of grapefruit juice, as this will prolong and amplify the effect. If it becomes too much for you to handle, take a glass of milk; it will kill the effect of the flush in a few minutes.

By March 2002, I had regained nearly all of my hearing about 8 weeks after the problem started. It seems as though the niacin did more than any other one thing; the rest was simply time to heal. I used a couple of different antibiotic eardrops the doctors prescribed for me the first week.

When I have a health problem, I firmly believe in doing anything and everything I can think of, all at the same time, to fix the problem as quickly as possible. Most people want to know exactly what worked---which of the modalities or supplements made the difference? I like to know as well, but to me it is more important to fix the problem as soon as possible, rather than figuring out specifically what did the trick.

I am into pleasure, not pain and suffering, yet I have endured enough pain and suffering for one lifetime. This time, I tried everything at once, but nothing seemed to be working. I have experienced many periods like this in the past with many problems, and always eventually found the right combination of treatments that work synergistically. Through prayer, I have always found that I woke up one morning and the problem is gone. That is the beauty of treating the whole body and letting the body heal itself. Treating a symptom, as most medical doctors do, is like taking an aspirin; the pain may go away for a while, but it doesn't fix the problem.

In 2011, a doctor told me that for every 7 years we spend abusing ourselves with bad eating habits, lack of sleep, smoking, drinking, and the many other things we do to tear down our bodies, our temple, it takes one year of doing everything right to allow the body to rebuild itself.

Learning to believe in yourself is just the first step. Then you start learning how to make the necessary changes that can make a difference in your life. Your health will follow as your determination increases and as your accomplishments grow day by day. You did not get into the condition you are in overnight, and you will not turn it around overnight. Be patient with yourself, but be determined to reverse each and every health issue, as only you can do this for yourself. Never forget that *Your Health is Your Choice.*

CHAPTER 9

Heart Attack

Removing blockages and rebuilding damage to my heart: In order to write this book, in January 2002, I moved to Bullhead City, Arizona, a small town about 100 miles south of Las Vegas (where I had lived for 60-plus years). This move took about 10 trips in my overloaded mini-truck. Every trip was a 12–16 hour day, and on my last trip, I noticed chest pains as I started to unload. I thought I had reversed all my health problems and could not imagine a heart problem happening to me, especially then, when I was feeling 30 years old.

I kept pushing myself, thinking, "I will work through it. It can't be my heart." However, the pains got worse and my pace became slower and slower. A couple of hours after dark, I surmised that it might be my heart, because I became nauseated and started sweating, and the pain was moving into my left shoulder. I had no phone in my house yet, and I was far enough out in the country that I did not have cell phone service, so I couldn't call for help. I didn't know where there was a hospital or even a fire department.

Fortunately, I had brought my ozone machine on this trip. I bagged up in my ozone bag and turned on the machine. Within an hour, the pain subsided and I was able to go to sleep. The pain was not overwhelming; if it had been, I would have tried to go to a hospital. Also, being in real denial, I was sure it could not be a heart attack. The pain was different from any I had experienced before, and I was extremely tired.

This all began on a Friday night. I made a mental note to get it checked out by a cardiologist as soon as I could, then spent the following 3 nights and 2 days in my ozone bag. I slept 10–12 hours each night and napped several times a day for 1–3 hours, never leaving the house.

Lying there in my ozone bag, I felt devastated and thought, “There goes my book. How could I possibly write a book about health and not be in perfect health myself?” I felt sorry for myself for several hours, when after a short prayer, the light came on. It became clear: “This is just another chapter.” I had 100 percent faith that God would guide me to the right people to reverse this problem, as he had with my many others. I realized this was just another opportunity to learn more about health, and all the stress went away.

While out of the ozone bag, I limited my physical activity quite a bit for the rest of the weekend and made adjustments in my diet until I figured out just what to do to correct this problem. Since I had had so much success using ozone with other health problems, it was the first thing that came to mind. My oxygen blood content had been down to 91 percent the first night I had the chest pains. This was the lowest reading I had ever taken on myself. That first night I slept 12 straight hours in the ozone bag; in the morning, 90 percent of my chest pains were gone and my oxygen blood level was 97 percent, a 1-point rise for every 2 hours in the bag.

My oximeter was one of the most difficult things I ever bought to help improve my health. When I first started using ozone, I was afraid of overuse and hurting myself, so I paid $900 for one just to be safe. I did use it a lot the first month (as described in Chapter 3), and then I finally realized that the blood can’t hold more than 100 percent, so I quit using it for a long time. The first time I really felt the need for it again was nearly 10 years later, and I was very thankful it was with me, enabling me to monitor my situation.

During my first heart attack, the tightness in my chest returned the second evening, so I checked my oxygen blood level again; it was down to 92 percent. This really surprised me, as I was still in denial about the link between the symptoms and my heart. Normally it would never drop more than 2–3 percent in a day unless I was really fighting a cold or was extremely run down. Even then, only once or twice in the past 5 years had it ever dropped 4 percent from morning to night.

The following Monday morning, I returned to Las Vegas and went directly to the Heart Institute of Nevada. The cardiologist, Dr. Morris, ran an EKG and discovered I had suffered a heart attack. More tests showed there was heart damage. The doctor's initial diagnosis was that I had an electrical short circuit caused by a blockage. He scheduled me for a complete examination, including blood work, 2 weeks later.

Meanwhile, he prescribed nitroglycerin, Coumadin, Ambien, and several other drugs. I still don't know what they were supposed to do. I was reluctant to take them, but I did not want to risk dying while waiting to see if my own protocol would work. The doctor assured me that dying was a definite possibility if I did not take the medication. I did as he had told me with the exception of the nitro, as I had no chest pains, and I only took half the amount of aspirin.

Over the following 7 days, I slept 9 to 10 hours a night in my ozone bag before my blood oxygen content rose up to 98–99 percent in the morning without dropping below 94 percent at night. This excessive use of the ozone burned my lungs, as noted in Chapter 3. Dr. Morris had given me NitroQuick to use when I had chest pains, but it was a couple of weeks before I needed one. Ozone kept the pain down to the point where I did not need one for the first week or two; but when I had to stop the ozone to allow my lungs to heal, it was good to have the drugs. This forced me to take 2 aspirin a day to thin my blood as ordered, along with Coumadin.

Years ago, when I first started ozone therapy, a major concern was overuse. I would wake up every hour or two and recheck my oxygen blood content. It took twenty to thirty nights before I could relax and feel safe sleeping straight through the night without repeating this process. In the past, spending two or three nights sleeping in the ozone bag to bring my oxygen blood level up to 98–99 percent eliminated all of my cold symptoms, and my very high energy level would return.

I had been overweight for many years; and when I retired, I was nonfunctional because of my many health challenges. My weight went up to 310 pounds before I got started on the process of learning to restore my health. I have tried different diets and have fasted many times, usually several days at a time, and on one occasion, for 30 days. Due to my firsthand experience, I am fully aware that diet alone can dramatically improve my health. However, I live to eat, and had once mistakenly thought I could cheat on my diet and eat anything as long as I compensated by taking the right supplements. My heart problem proved me wrong. Therefore, I addressed it through diet first.

Magnetic therapy also helped my heart. On a second trip back to Las Vegas from Bullhead City, just a few days after my first heart attack, I began having chest pains again. I was about an hour away from help, which added to my concern, since I had not taken a nitro pill yet and had no idea what to expect from one. See chapter 4 to understand just what I did.

On my next trip back to Las Vegas, having forgotten my nitro pills once again, I began to have chest pains at about the same spot. Anxiety set in, my heart raced, and my chest hurt. I applied the magnets again with the same positive results. I never go anywhere without my magnets, but now I do not go anywhere without my nitro either. I feel it is foolish not to be prepared for everything and anything.

A quick outline of my plan to address my heart problem:

1. Diet first: I changed to 80 percent fresh raw fruits and vegetables. For a more in-depth understanding of this, see Chapter 13 on nutrition and the importance of a balanced pH.

2. Ozone, holding a pillow or towel under my chin and around my throat to reduce leakage.

3. Exercise: This is very crucial to health, yet difficult when one is not up to par. See Chapter 12 on exercise and rebounding

4. Chelation: I used both IV and oral chelation. See Chapter 2 for more information.

5. Magnets: as described above.

Caution: Do not keep these magnets in place for more than 20 minutes at a time, but you can repeat it several times a day. I used them because I had no ozone available the first time, and the second time I was taking a break from using ozone due to burned lungs.

I had not realized the relationship between my teeth, my gum infection, an ear infection, and my heart problem. Not one of the several MDs suggested there could be a connection to my teeth, and none of the 4 dentists I had gone to over the past several months had mentioned I could have complications that might lead to other health problems. Most of the MDs and dentists who have treated me were so absorbed in their specific field of expertise that they do not see the whole health picture. They focus on treating symptoms of the body's imbalance while allowing harmful bacteria to flourish and evolve into different health problems, depending on each patient's weaknesses.

I continued to use ozone every night (except for the couple of weeks after I burned my lungs, as noted). As long as my oxygen level remained over 95 percent or higher, I had no chest pains. However, when it dropped to 94, I felt minor chest pains; 93 percent started to scare me. It only went down to 93 percent a couple of times since this started, and the drop was associated with fast fluctuation in blood oxygen levels (which I have yet been unable to understand).

A friend suggested I might be low in iron, which is necessary to hold oxygen in the blood. Another friend said she had been using an oxygen tank for over a year, but that after taking Seasilver for 2 weeks, she was completely off the tank. Two of her friends were also able to do this. I had tried several bottles in the past with no noticeable benefit, but had no apparent health problem at the time. I began taking both Seasilver and iron after my heart attack, and I did feel some benefit. Since the FDA took Seasilver off the market soon after, I didn't get the chance to try it long enough to say for sure whether it worked or not.

When I review my notes of everything taking place at that time, I now realize that my teeth were undoubtedly the underlying problem. It did not occur to me then, as I had no pain or noticeable problem. The iron and Seasilver did help to keep my oxygen level up, but I still shouldn't have needed so much time in the ozone bag.

Since it takes 2 hours in the ozone bag to raise my blood oxygen level by 1 percent, I had my machine custom fitted for adding an oxygen tank to reduce the time needed. When ozone is made from oxygen instead of ambient air, the percentage of ozone is much higher. I hooked in the small tank and regulator and turned the machine on low. Within 1 hour, the tank was empty, but it brought my oxygen level up 2 percent. My blood oxygen level had increased much faster than I expected, but the time and money it cost to refill the small tank was not worth the time saved in the bag.

Thinking that my insurance company would cover oxygen, I went back to the cardiologist to get a prescription. The doctor told me that insurance would not pay for supplemental oxygen unless my blood oxygen level was below 90 percent much of the time. It is difficult to believe they would not help keep a person as healthy as possible to prevent future damage to his or her heart. I couldn't afford to pay for the oxygen, so I continued spending 8 to 10 hours a night in the ozone bag.

After several days of trying to keep my oxygen blood level up and having chest pains when it dropped, I went back to the cardiologist. He wanted to admit me into the hospital for a few days to monitor me. I asked if I could take my ozone machine and he said he did not think the hospital would like that. I told him I would not go without it, because I believed it would eliminate my blockages; he did not push it any further.

Finally, I called my friend Dr. Bonlie for suggestions on keeping my oxygen level elevated. He said that my burned lungs were not allowing enough oxygen transfer with normal breathing. He recommended stopping the ozone until my lungs healed and using an oxygen bottle for supplemental oxygen. He also suggested that I consider taking DMSA as a supplemental oral chelation to help clear the blockages in my circulatory system. I did follow his suggestions, and they were very helpful to me.

Problems with my teeth had started 6 months earlier, and now I am more certain than ever that my teeth were partially, if not entirely, responsible for my heart attacks. The cardiologist was correct that blockages caused the attacks, but the infection brought them on sooner than if I had not had it.

I had just had a third tooth pulled a few days before my heart problem started, and I was certain I had an infection present. The dentist had told me I did not need antibiotics, and he would not give me any. At the time, I was not aware of any infection, so I didn't push it.

By the time I called Dr. Bonlie, I was sure I was getting an infection. He told me to go back to my dentist, insist on a prescription for antibiotics, and to discontinue using the magnet on my teeth. He said it would draw my body's reserve healing energy to the area of my teeth, but that my heart needed it more.

After taking the antibiotic and the DMSA that he suggested, all of these problems disappeared. I felt 100 percent better right away and was able to get back to working in my yard and building my patio. I had to work at a much slower pace than before, as I still had the heart damage to repair. Within a couple of weeks, I was able to cut the ozone back to 4–5 hours every other night.

My friend and one of my dentists, Dr. Donald Brown, DDS, understand the inner relationship between our life force (meridians) and our health. He told me there is little doubt in his mind that the infection and the subsequent loss of three teeth could have precipitated my heart attacks.

At the Heart Institute of Nevada, I was tested again to see if my heart had improved. The doctor compared current photos with those from 3 months earlier. There was no doubt that my heart was worse than before. His urgency in scheduling an angiogram scared me, and he pushed me very hard to do an angioplasty. As had Dr. Morris, this doctor assured me that nothing would clear the blockages except an angioplasty on both arteries, which would last a couple of years; then I would need another. After 2 or 3, I would require bypass surgery: that is the life I could expect. He assured me that both arteries would only get worse and nothing could change that because of my age.

I am so thankful that I followed my instincts, as I love feeling 20 years old; I am sure now that I will never need to do any of the things the cardiologists told me would be necessary.

This time when he suggested doing an angiogram, I was much more receptive. He scheduled it for 6:00 a.m. the following morning. Three months earlier, I had been sure I would not need one because I was certain that the ozone oral and IV chelation had eliminated the blockages, but they appeared not to have worked. I had been sure three months would be enough time to clean my arteries, but the photographs showed that my heart damage was not better; it was worse than before, convincing me and filling me with fear and doubt.

When I had the angiogram, I was very surprised to find that I actually had no significant blockages remaining. I realize now that I shouldn't have been surprised. I have reversed dozens of my own health problems myself. I feel certain there is no health problem that cannot be overcome with God's help. The doctors had me convinced that I had no choice but to let them do what they felt was right. I wondered how many people they had killed just by making people believe only they could save them.

I was sorry the doctor would not take the time to see the exit wound in my leg from the angiogram. I put the negative field of a neodymium magnet on that spot as soon as the tube came out; an hour later there had been no bleeding, bruising, swelling, or redness. Two of the nurses were so impressed that they wanted my phone number so they could learn more about magnetic therapy and for a source to buy magnets.

Once again I was able to work 10–12 hours a day, just not as hard or as fast. I was 100 percent sure I would be able to restore my heart completely and get back to a normal life. I don't believe there is such a thing as irreversible damage to any part of the body, with the possible exception of a brain injury. There is a lot of research on brain damage that looks promising, and it is quite likely in the near future that even brain damage could be repaired. (I wrote this part of the book in 2002.)

I had hoped the doctor would keep an open mind and not think of my recovery as a miracle but rather give credit to my methods. While it may be a miracle, I believe the doctors can (and need to) learn how they can better help their patients by using these methods on anyone and everyone they treat in the future.

At this point in my life, I believe doctors are very important for medical testing. They tell us how serious our condition is, give us options to keep us alive, and assist us in finding solutions. I do not believe a doctor should ever tell us there is no hope. I do not believe we will get better once our minds accept that as fact, because the mind is very powerful over the body, mind, and spirit. When I hear someone talking about the placebo effect and dismissing it like it is insignificant, it amazes me. How can any intelligent person not realize the power of the mind? It is the most important thing we have. Science hasn't begun to understand the mind's potential. Once we learn to harness its power, we will be able to heal ourselves of all sickness and disease spontaneously, without the need for outside intervention.

It worked out well that a doctor friend could schedule me early in May 2002, for 2 weeks of experimental magnetic therapy for his research. I left for Canada just a few days after the angiogram confirmed that all of my heart blockages were gone.

On my trip, I had chest pains and had to take nitro. The anxiety of the trip was really getting to me and brought on my chest pains far more than the physical exertion of travel. A short time later, I took 2 more nitro pills because of the increased pain. I hadn't taken any at all over the past month.

Once I arrived and could feel the relaxing effects of the magnetic energy passing through my body. I believed this allowed my body's immune system to accelerate my healing so much that after 12-1/2 hours, I felt so good, I discontinued all of my medication. Now I was only taking spirulina, wheat-grass, rice bran, and some protein powder. These are the most nutrient-dense foods in the world that I am aware of; between them, they cover the full spectrum of all the known nutrients the body needs. These are all whole foods, so any nutrients that haven't yet been discovered are likely to be found in them. (I have learned a lot more since I wrote this in 2002, but I still take all of those supplements. I have additional information in Chapter 13.)

On the second day, I walked about a mile to a super Wal-Mart to pick up some things. By the end of the day, I was so sure I would get a 100 percent improvement in my heart muscle; I called my cardiologist to set an appointment as soon as I got back to redo all of my tests.

I returned to Las Vegas in just 9 days, feeling 30 years younger. I have said that I now feel 20 years old, but actually, I feel even better. When I was in my twenties, I was drunk all night and sick all day, so I didn't know what it was like to feel absolutely fantastic.

When someone asks me, "How are you today?" I say, "Just purt' near perfect;" and I often follow that with "if I felt any better, I couldn't stand myself." I love feeling 20 years old with the same weight and waist size I had then. It comes from understanding just how simple health can be.

Instantly stopping heart attacks and bleeding:

Learn to use cayenne pepper and its tincture.

I have heard too many doctors at health trade shows claim that cayenne pepper really works well for me not to believe it. Dr. Christopher and his colleague, Dr. Richard Schulz, have been stating for over 50 years that cayenne pepper can reduce heart disease dramatically. The answers have been here for many years; but the AMA, FDA, and pharmaceutical industry have been so successful in convincing our population that only the MDs they train are capable of deciding how to treat disease and what is best for us.

Note: If you want to learn more about this subject, you can Google information on both doctors above. They both have written many books, and this subject is covered extensively. You can also go to www.YourHealthisYourChoice.org *and look for media in the lower left of the home page and find archived conference calls. Look for the ones with my friend, Phil Fans; he is a 90-year-old scientist with amazing stories about health. He is still an active teacher at a college in Utah, and he explains the many benefits of cayenne and reveals some secrets about cancer and heart disease.*

I carried a bottle of the tincture in my pocket for 2 years after my 3 heart attacks; but fortunately, I've never had the need to use it. Because I had been so successful in cleansing my circulatory system with chelation, ozone, and magnetic therapy, I haven't had a problem with my heart since. After going through my notes and writing this, this morning I put my computer to sleep and went to Whole Foods to buy a bottle of cayenne tincture; I will start carrying it again just in case someone needs it.

I believe the world has a right to know, and that the FDA and AMA should be disseminating this type of information to our nation. It is important to learn what we can do for ourselves, our families, and everyone around us.

How to survive a heart attack when you are alone: This article will be posted on my website, www.DRhealthclub.com. And look for my e-book, *Your Health is Your Choice: Health Made Simple*, on my website, www.YourHealthisYourChoice.ORG

CHAPTER 10

Feet: Stopping the pain

Most of my life I have suffered with excessively hot feet and, more recently, very painful plantar fascia; yet I have overcome both problems. If you think you may have this problem, I would highly recommend taking a look at the Mayo Clinic website, www.mayoclinic.com/health/plantar-fasciitis/DS00508.

Plantar fasciitis (PLAN-turfas-e-I-tis) involves pain and inflammation of a thick band of tissue, called the *plantar fascia*, which runs across the bottom of the foot.

In 1962, I burned my feet while working a brush fire. I had second and third-degree burns and was off work for over a month. From then on, my feet have felt excessively hot most of the time. This problem has become progressively worse and has caused me to lose thousands of hours of sleep.

To sleep at night, I have needed a fan blowing on my feet, or a wet towel on them, or sometimes both. I have asked many doctors over the past 50 years about this problem. Most of them never had a patient with this complaint or have never heard of the problem. The few who had anything at all to say about it said that it was psychosomatic, and that I needed to learn to live with it. I did, but many times the discomfort became almost unbearable. I had pretty well accepted that it was psychosomatic, having never heard of anyone else with this problem.

Around the year 2000, a friend of mine overheard a woman working at a health food store recommend alpha lipoic acid to another customer. He called me from Florida to tell me about this.

My friend told me the woman had recommended using 250 milligrams of the NOW brand, twice a day. After trying three stores in Las Vegas and not finding that brand, I got a bottle of MRM brand in 300-milligram pills. I went to a movie a few hours later after I took my first pill. My feet were so hot during the movie that I took off my shoes and socks and set my bare feet on the cold concrete floor, as I was so uncomfortable I couldn't enjoy the movie. I took another before going to bed; I still used a fan but the discomfort was less noticeable the next day.

By the 5th day, I felt about a 20 to 25 percent improvement. I slept that night with a fan on low instead of high and woke up a couple of times with my feet under the covers. My feet must have become cold, and I unconsciously covered them while sleeping.

Each time I woke up, my feet felt hot, and I would uncover them, then fall back to sleep in just a couple of minutes. When I woke up in the morning, my feet felt cold. This was very unusual. They would only feel cold when I put them in cold water or if I was outside in very cold weather.

I called my friend in Florida to tell him of my progress and asked if he could compare it with that of the person who told him about this treatment. He reported that the person had said he noticed a big improvement in the first week and that the problem was totally under control within a month.

Ten days after taking alpha lipoic acid, I felt a 40 to 50 percent improvement, and for the first time in several years, I went to bed with cold feet. One hour later, I woke up and my feet were very warm, but not hot. I put the fan on low and went back to sleep within a few minutes. I woke up the next morning with my feet comfortably under the covers. I also had not had any noticeable discomfort with hot feet during the day for several days.

I felt certain this protocol would fix the problem by at least 80 percent within a few more weeks. It turned out that I hit a plateau and went several months with no noticeable improvement. I ended up going to Florida to work on this book, and the first thing I did was to go to the health food store where my friend got the information. It turns out that I was using less than half the amount I should have been. I bought the brand they recommended, and with a few more days of the proper amount of the right product, I have seldom needed to use a fan since.

Sore feet

My plantar fasciitis started in 2001 while helping a friend with his company; the work kept me up on my feet 16 to 18 hours a day. After about 2 months, walking became very painful. I tried orthopedic shoes and arch supports, and I went to several podiatrists, but nothing helped.

A doctor used a combination of 30-minute far-infrared heat lamp treatments and B12 shots twice a week; these seemed to help a little, but the benefit didn't last long. I gave up after a couple of months and looked all over again for a more lasting way to address this very painful problem.

I finally tried a pair of Nikken Mag Steps and felt some relief. I had tried Nikken magnetic products in the past and found that they did work, but only for a short time, as they have both positive and negative fields against the skin. This is another case where the product helped a lot at first, but benefits reduced when it was used continuously for a couple of weeks.

Then I tried a Mannatech product in powder form called Ambrotose. It contains 2 essential sugar molecules that we do not get in our normal diet. It reportedly helps repair damaged DNA, which allows cells to replicate correctly. I used one bottle of this powder, and all the pain went away. This benefit lasted for more than a year before my feet started bothering me again. However, I refused to deal with the person in my up line again, (Mannatech is a multilevel-marketing company) and they would not let me move under another person so I started looking for other products.

At a health trade show in Las Vegas, I met Dr. Luke from the American Herbal Laboratories in Rosemead, California. He has a computer-generated test of meridians that prints results showing the weaknesses in various organs. Several others had already tested me with much more expensive machines, and I wanted to see how this compared. To my surprise, all the tests I got at that trade show were very close in diagnosing my health issues. Of course, none of them wanted to claim their machine did diagnosis because of the FDA, but they all provided me with an idea of my personal health weaknesses. I learned what supplements were necessary to maintain and improve my health.

I told Dr. Luke about my foot problems and pain, about them being very hot, and about the improvement I had had with the alpha lipoic acid. He made notes about my use of the ALA, possibly to recommend it to other patients. He then prescribed an herbal nutritional supplement and told me to take one capsule twice a day.

The good news was that my feet were pain free for the first time in more than a year. The pain went away completely within 5 days. Dr. Luke's supplement was very expensive; but since it worked, it was worth it.

He also gave me another herbal supplement, Male Plus, for my kidney stress. He said it would also strengthen my heart and improve my sex life. I cannot say for sure whether it worked for my kidneys and heart, but there is no doubt that there was a difference in my sex life (or at least sexual desire). I discussed that in Chapter 6; it was slow coming back, even with this new product, but there was a noticeable improvement.

As of 2011, the improvement in my feet had lasted for nearly 10 years, although in the past few they have bothered me from time to time. They get hot some nights, requiring me to use a fan once again, but the increase in my sex drive was short lived.

I lost track of Dr. Luke and really wish I could find him, as I have told many people about him but now do not know how to get them in touch. This is one of the most important reasons I feel everyone should keep a log of their health issues, the severity of each, and what helps and what does not help. I had forgotten about using ALA for my hot feet several years ago when the problem went away. Now this minor problem has come back subtly and I will start taking it again. I hope to see the same benefits.

In 2005, I started taking an enzyme product called Vitalzym that made a real difference. I found out that all cellular repairs are done with enzymes, and I believe Vitalzym has one of the most complete formulations.

Enzymes need a combination of things to do their job. Minerals are the foundation of life. Without their presence in a balanced, assumable form, the foundation cannot be laid. I have been aware of this for about 20 years and have searched for the best of the best for nearly 15 years. I believe I have finally found it: Trace Minerals and Mag/Cal, a 1/3 calcium and 2/3 magnesium combination. (Both are distributed by A2Z Health Products.)

Enzymes then need amino acids to build on the foundation of minerals. There are 22 different types; 8 are essential, meaning that we must get them from what we eat. The body can make the rest, if it is provided with the right nutrients. (Most of us don't eat a well-balanced diet that provides all the needed nutrients, so supplementing is necessary to maintain long-term health.) These 22 amino acids make about 50,000 combinations of nutrients the body needs. If you are missing just one essential amino acid, you could be missing thousands of repair possibilities; these are so vast that science has only become aware of them. We have very little understanding of how each of these combinations works.

There is also a need for water, oxygen, magnetic energy, and other types of energy that science knows very little about at this time. Only in recent years have there been devices made that are capable of even measuring them. Here is the point: when you try to break down all the microbiology, health can become very complicated.

I like to try to keep things simple, like walking into a room, flipping on a switch, and there is light. I don't need to understand all there is to know about electricity to enjoy the light.

Health can be just that simple as well; the underlying cause of nearly all health issues is some form of pathogen or environmental toxin that disturbs function at the cellular level. Sodium Chlorite

(MMS) addresses nearly all of them to some degree. Sodium Chlorite (MMS), when mixed with citric acid, creates chlorine dioxide. It is very inexpensive and can "turn your light on" with most health problems; it is just that simple.

I cannot say how much a part Sodium Chlorite (MMS) played in relieving my foot problem, but until I started using MMS in February 1997, I was not pain free. Everything I did helped in some degree to educate me far more than I expected would be necessary to get beyond the pain. I learned not only far more than I had expected to, but far more than I thought I was capable of. It has all been worth it. Now I am 100 percent pain free and can walk for miles with no foot pain at all. I still take the enzymes, the minerals, and other supplements, as I do not want to go backwards with my health ever again.

With determination to find the answers and through knowledge, it is simple. Prayer will bring you the answers you need to change your life, your health, and all that you need to enjoy the love and life we share; as we are all one with God.

CHAPTER 11

Health made simple: All health starts with cleansing!

Only the body can heal itself. It is up to us to cleanse, detoxify, eat properly, and exercise so the immune system can do its job. Pure water is also essential to detoxing and maintaining optimum health.

All health starts with cleansing and detoxing to eliminate the toxins that overwhelm our immune system. Parasites, fungus, molds, liver and gall bladder stones, many harmful chemicals, metals, and environmental toxins plague our bodies. I have experienced miracles in my life and health through internal cleansing.

We have 10 vital organs and/or organ systems that we need to consider when beginning a cleansing program. It is very important that cleanses are done in proper order, or we run the risk of detoxing one organ but overwhelming another. This could cause a serious illness that may trigger needless pain and suffering, not to mention the loss of time and money. Anyone who does not conduct a cleansing program will probably experience physical sickness often throughout life.

If you face mental and physical hardships, stick with your cleanse and ride out the storm. The results are worth it. Make sure to clue in your family and loved ones about what to expect; otherwise, they will surely try to talk you out of following through with it. Tell them about your health goals and share what your body experiences during this process.

You should get started today. Cleansing is not very expensive. I highly recommend Dr. Hulda Clark's books, *A Cure for All Cancer* and *A Cure for All Disease*. She meticulously explains how, why, and when to do each cleanse and provides a list of sources to buy what is needed for each.

Dr. Clark recommends this order of cleanses:

- Colon
- Liver and gallbladder
- Parasite
- Kidney and bladder
- Heart and cholesterol
- Brain
- Blood
- Glands and prostate
- Eyes
- Skin

Cleanse and Detox

We are filters. The body must filter everything we breathe, eat, drink, or absorb through the skin. Ideally, the body assimilates nutrients and eliminates contaminants. When a filter becomes full of pollutants and contaminants, it is of no further value. It seems obvious that the cleaner our filtering system, the healthier we will stay. With frequent cleansing, our bodies will last longer, just like when we change the oil filter in our cars. Most gas engines start having problems around 100,000 miles and a few last 150,000. I know a few people who are still driving cars with 300,000 miles on them, because they change the oil regularly and take good care of the car. I believe we can do the same with our bodies. I do not feel anywhere near middle aged, even though I am 70.

Most of my life, I have lived to eat and have eaten anything I wanted whenever the urge hit. For me to continue to do this, I must cleanse my organs often. I believe we can put just about anything into our bodies that we want to if we know how to get contaminants out. However, I don't believe that anyone living today knows how to cleanse all contaminants; the list of toxins seems to be growing every day. It is smarter and easier to eat what we know is good for us and to stay away from what is unhealthy.

If any one of us did not shower daily, I'm sure we could tell. However, what if someone had never cleansed their insides? Do you think we could tell? Yes, of course we could. Such a person would be sick and tired all the time, rarely feel good, and would have chronic headaches, sore throats, colds, and flu. The colon would be impacted with old fecal matter and would be a breeding ground for parasites, fungus, and harmful bacteria, as well as a permanent hiding place for toxins and carcinogens.

Eliminating harmful waste from our organs, colon, and cells is exciting, especially when many are large enough to see. When I did the parasite cleanse, it eliminated hundreds of parasites large enough to see in my stools. Some were several inches long and others were small, but there was no doubt they were parasites. According to what I have read about cleansing, I am sure it eliminated millions of microscopic parasites at the same time.

Cleansing and detoxifying go hand and hand. Most cleanses address toxicity at the same time as they rid our body of waste. When I did the liver and gallbladder cleanse, I filled a quart jar full of gallstones and liver stones. I am sure there were more than 2,000 of them—maybe 3,000.

Several years prior to doing this cleanse, I was diagnosed with a hiatal hernia. I had heartburn so bad I could not sleep lying down for 2 or 3 years. The acid would come up into my throat and wake me. Even when I watched what I ate, I still needed many different types of antacids each night. Three doctors wanted to operate on me for this problem. After a 6-day liver and gallbladder cleanse, I never had heartburn again. This is just one of numerous benefits I have received from different types of cleanses.

Whether purchasing products from a health food store, a friend, or a neighbor, please make sure they are all made from natural whole food sources when possible. Using all natural products is the best way to quickly get on the road to better health. By far, the majority of products on the market today do not come from natural whole food sources, even though they say they do. Our body cannot assimilate many of their listed ingredients.

It is a good idea to become friends with someone at a health food store who knows what the best types of nutrients are. Ask about the difference between calcium carbonate and calcium citrate. Calcium carbonate is a rock-source mineral and calcium citrate is a plant-source mineral. The plant source is always better assimilated by our bodies. If the person does not give the correct answer, find someone else to help you, and make another new friend.

Remember, when we are looking for that special person to help us through the maze of products, they are all trying to sell us something. Most of us can't afford to buy everything. I know dozens of people in the health field, and many are very knowledgeable, but most will not admit when they do not know what to recommend for our specific problem. I have often gone to several places asking for recommendations and advice, but usually I will not buy anything until I get opinions from two or three people and understand the product. This is also an opportunity to get to know a lot of people in the health and wellness field. We then can better determine who is in it just for the money or who is there for the love of it and really wants to help others.

I have researched many sources for products of the highest quality, only to be disappointed either to find they did not work or that it was not a completely natural product as advertised. I have fanatically searched out products that are organically grown or wild harvested, and made sure the plants were never sprayed with chemical fertilizers, pesticides, or herbicides. I am committed to finding the absolute finest quality products for my health.

Getting started with cleansing

I recommend that you write down everything you eat and drink for 2 weeks, along with the time of day. Include the times of your bowel movements. You should have one within 2 hours of each meal.

The goal is to improve your bowel transition time. You improve your diet by eating more fruits and vegetables and less meat, sugars and starches. Fish, if chewed well, can take as little as 2 hours to digest; chicken takes longer, and red meat can take 8 to 24 hours or even longer if not chewed well.

Be exact in your journal when recording your progress, as many improvements are subtle, and you may overlook them if you are not keeping careful records of the below:

1. What you ate, time, and date ______________________________

   ____

   ____

2. Time and date of each bowel movement ___________________

   ____

   ____

3. If you are having a urinary issue, list what you drink and the time and date of each elimination. ________________________

   ____

   ____

4. Your general well-being. List all aches and pains, any symptoms of ailment, and any medical diagnoses. ________

   ____

   ____

5. Frequency and intensity of head and body aches. Rate intensity on a scale of 1 to 10. ______________________

____

____

____

6. Nausea. ______________________________________

____

____

7. Energy level. __________________________________

____

____

____

8. Any other illnesses (colds, flu, etc.) ________________

____

____

____

9. General mental state. Rate the following on a 1 to 10 scale of intensity and note how long they last:

   a. amount of depression __________________________

   ____

   b. anger, frustration, exhaustion ___________________

   ____

   c. energy level ________________________________

   ____

   ____

Maintaining this journal once a day will help you start on your road to better health more than any other single thing you do. Write down your thoughts and feelings and any other things that influence your day.

- Your success depends entirely on your determination, as no one can do this for you.

Many people experience a "healing crisis" while they are cleansing. Here are some helpful hints:

6. For nausea, drink ginger tea or add fresh ginger root from the health food store to your salad. You can also grate ginger. Don't heat it over 105 degrees.
7. Depression can often be helped with a magnesium supplement. Dr. Philpot has used magnets very successfully. In his handbook on bio magnetics, he says to place the negative pole of a small magnet over each temple.

More to consider:

Do you know that CO_2 is one of the body's main waste products? Yes, carbon dioxide! Do you know what makes that soda or beer bubbly? Of course you do; it's CO_2. Now think about this the next time you open that soda can: it's like drinking your own urine! Do you think it will taste as good? Visualization is an important key to success in changing eating habits to maintain good health. So the next time you think you want a carbonated drink, visualize someone in a bottling plant peeing in every bottle. (This is not to be taken literally, as there are many books explaining the health benefits of drinking your own urine. It is a visualization exercise to help you stop drinking carbonated beverages. To my knowledge, there is little to no benefit in drinking them.)

Anything we understand seems simple, and health seems simple to me today!

Our own unique life experiences give us the opportunity to share with one another for mutual benefit. Those who are inspired to learn how to improve our quality of life benefit us all. Many people have taken advantage of the opportunity to participate in my conference calls (held every Tuesday evening at 5:45 to 8:00 p.m. PST). I host and handle them just like I did my radio show. Many people have learned a great deal about health by listening and asking questions of the exceptional health care professionals I interview. The calls are live and interactive by phone. You can also listen to the recordings archived on the Internet and hear many remarkable healers, doctors, and spiritual beings sharing knowledge and what they feel are the most important lessons of their lives. You can find the information to participate in the calls posted on the following websites: www.YourHealthisYourChoice.org, www.DRhealthClub.com, and www.A2ZhealthProducts.com.

We can expand our own knowledge by taking advantage of these remarkable experiences to improve our health and our lives. Many of my experiences are pieces of the puzzle of understanding how to use the energy we all have access to, which Christ used to heal the sick and give sight to the blind. I am inspired to learn just what Christ meant when he said, "The least among you can do all that I have done and even greater things."

I also want to address Optimum D-Tox, made from the *Schidigera Yucca*, a plant that grows wild in the Mojave Desert. It has many nutritional health benefits and incredible cleansing properties. It stimulates the endocrine system to balance hormones naturally. Yucca helps to detox the colon and provides many micronutrients.

My current clothing size and weight are the same as when I got out of the Marine Corps when I was 20, and I did this without dieting or exercise, beyond rebounding fifteen minutes a day.

On YouTube (search under "DennisRichardBooks," and "MMSdr1"), I have several videos of James Slone, a PhD in nutrition, and me, which explain how and why this works as it does. In addition, I have a short video on how I mix Sodium Chlorite (MMS) and use it for brushing and flossing my teeth, along with many other videos.

I have heard many doctors say that fungus and yeast are the underlying cause of 70 to 80 percent of America's health problems. I first heard this in 2006. Dr. William Hitt, a nearly 80 year old MD, was the first one that took the time to explain that to me.

After seeing 6 doctors in Las Vegas who performed thousands of dollars' worth of tests on me, none could come up with any reasons for why I was feeling so bad. I went to see Dr. Hitt and Dr. Humiston at the Hitt Center in Tijuana. It just took him a few hours to evaluate my tests and tell me that the most likely problem was fungus and yeast, *Candida* being the worst.

I took some ozone treatments (see Chapter 3), and I left with Dr. Humiston's Candida Kit, a large bag filled with 3 months' supply of herbs. Within 2 months, I felt like a new person and continued for another month. By then I lost 30 pounds, along with all cravings and the desire to eat, if I was not actually hungry. Dr. Humiston has made available his Candida kit and information and it is available on his website, www.candidamd.com

The diet was a little tough at first, because it was limited to many things I normally did not eat at that time (a lot of vegetables and just a small amount of meat). I was to have no sweets, cheese, and dairy of any type, pasta, wheat, or fermented things that feed fungus. Drinking only water, and a lot of it, for the 3 months was what it took to get it all behind me. I felt amazing and would drive 350 miles once a month just for the opportunity to talk to these doctors. They were both very kind and always took time to speak with me and answer all of my questions, of which I always had many.

This is the only doctor's office whose waiting room I have ever looked forward to sitting in—for the chance to talk to other patients and listen to their stories. Many had nothing but hope, as doctors in the States had told them their illnesses were terminal and that nothing could be done. I spoke with many who had been told in the United States that their days were numbered; they came back to this office 10 and even 20 years later just for checkups.

Talking to dozens of people there, I heard about the Hoxey Clinic in Tijuana and went there many times just for the education.

Again, I found the doctors all working from their hearts for far less than they could make elsewhere, but they had the satisfaction of doing what was right for their patients without the restrictions placed on them by the FDA and the AMA, which are under the control of big pharmaceutical companies.

In 2008, I met nutripath, Dr. Sal D'Onofrio; he wrote *Yeast Control in Seven Days*. It was written in layman's language and is intended to help anyone who is interested in wellness using natural health principles. "Wellness through Education" is his motto. He wrote his book because of the lack of literature offering a quick, effective, safe, and understandable method of dealing with Candida. Candida Albicans is a fungus, a form of yeast that is a normal inhabitant of the large intestine. Candida is not pathogenic when balanced with other types of friendly flora, maintaining an internal environment that allows all the microorganisms to work in harmony. Candida itself is not the problem; an imbalanced digestive system affects the body's ability to metabolize nutrients, which leads to blood sugar imbalances, parasites, and allergies associated with Candida.

Dr. D'Onofrio is among the most knowledgeable doctors I have ever met in his understanding of how to support the body's needs to heal itself. He is a very spiritual person who really works from his heart with all of his patients, giving them his time and educating them on what they can do for themselves. He has been kind enough to spend a lot of time teaching me many things. He even proofed my book to make sure I do not give any misleading information in my effort to share the things that have helped me overcome my many health issues.

His book emphasizes the importance of internal cleansing and balancing the internal terrain that supports the body's immune system. I highly recommend that everyone read it and his other book, *The Digestible Digest*, as well. They really help to make health seem simple. They are available at www.healthguardians.com.

The Power of Positive Thinking is Useful in Several Ways!

Stay focused on your goals: Remember that we are 70 to 80 percent water. At my body weight, I am about 16 gallons of water; and I drink about that much water every 3 weeks. It makes sense that every 3 weeks my body's water supply is completely replenished. If my math is correct, we are approximately 75 percent renewed every 2 weeks. Our blood is mostly water, and science tells us that every blood cell is 100 percent replaced every 4 months. We get a completely new set of cells every 7 years. One of the most important things to improve our health is to drink a lot of pure water.

Visualization: Visualize all the bad guys packing up and leaving as your bad blood cells die off. Visualize your body becoming stronger and healthier as your lymph system and your elimination system clean every cell in your body. Visualization can be very helpful in your healing process. Think about this: everything ever invented, created, or even accomplished started with an idea—a thought, which then became a dream, a plan, and then reality.

I think we get energy from our two most valuable sources: our sun's 6,400 Kelvin light spectrum color vibrational frequencies, which allow a type of photosynthesis to take place in the body, and the earth's magnetic field, which produces a different type of energy frequency. My friend, Adam Abraham, explained the concept of sun gazing to me just a few months ago. Another very close friend, Ed, has been trying to get me to walk barefoot in the grass for close to 30 years to help ground me. Doing them both together has just recently become a compulsion of mine (I can't say it has made a difference, as I have only been doing it for a short time). Because my expectations are high, I feel it will help me mentally and physically, and quite likely, spiritually. I spend about 15 to 20 minutes each morning in prayer and meditation, experiencing "being in the moment" and the warmth of the sun. This, along with releasing emotional energy blockages, has allowed me to be 100 percent free of anxiety.

I believe my experiences outlined in this book can really help you make ***Your Health Your Choice.***

CHAPTER 12

Exercise

No need to break a sweat. The easiest and most efficient form of exercise that anyone can do is rebounding. As noted earlier, a rebounder is a small trampoline. Jumping on it exercises every cell in the body simultaneously. It can help us to obtain optimum health without risking injury. You can start a minute at a time if that is all you can do. You will be amazed how fast you can work up to 15 minutes a day. When I first started, it hurt so much I didn't think I could do it at all.

I compare jumping on a rebounder with the action of a 2-stroke single-piston engine. The down stroke increases the G-force on every cell at once. This helps each one excrete its waste, leaving a small vacuum at the top of the stroke, aiding the cell in its intake of nutrients. In addition, the stress of the down stroke strengthens cells. It is a great form of exercise for the whole body.

The lymph system is the vacuum cleaner of the body and is critical to maintaining good health. We have more lymph fluid than blood. We all know the blood carries life-giving nutrients and oxygen to each cell, and that the heart drives it through the circulatory system. The lymph fluid picks up cellular waste, dead cells, toxins, and carcinogens and carries them out of the body.

Once I better understood the importance and benefits of moving the lymph fluid (which can only be achieved with motion through a series of one-way valves), I bought a sit-down rebounder as it hurt too much to stand up and jump. I would sit in front of the TV and bounce up and down for a minute or two, and then I would rest for a few minutes. Within a couple of weeks, I was bouncing for 15 minutes without a break. I then moved up to a mini trampoline and set it in front of the TV. Within a few weeks, I was able to rebound on that, too, for 15 minutes.

Bodily pain comes primarily from two things: toxic buildup and the lack of oxygen at the cellular level. Rebounding addresses both. The motion removes the toxins through the lymph system, gets us breathing deeper (more oxygen), and stimulates the heart to beat faster. It is very important to drink a lot of water before and after exercising to flush out toxins.

Jumping also separates every vertebra in the spine and every joint in the body, knees, and legs. This allows toxins to be cleared out and new lymph fluid in to help lubricate each joint. If you feel rebounding is too painful, go slowly. The pain will soon go away. Within a few days, I felt so much better. Within a few weeks, I found myself looking forward to doing it.

The 4 main benefits of rebounding are that it:

1. Moves lymph fluid to cleanse each cell.

2. Eliminates waste at the cellular level.

3. Strengthens cells.

4. Lubricates joints.

Now that I know the importance of exercise, I still prefer not to break a sweat. It's not that I don't believe sweating is good for us and helps cleanse our internal body. It's just that I believe we can maintain our health with exercise that doesn't overstress the body unless our goal is to be a body builder, weight lifter, or professional athlete. Most of us have a hard time maintaining a proper pH balance in our blood because of the foods we eat. Most people seem to believe that over exercising is necessary to maintain health, but it really just adds more acid to our systems, making it more difficult to maintain a balanced blood pH. The harder we exercise the more lactic acid we create.

By no means am I a fitness expert. I maintain very good health and fitness even while limiting my exercise to primarily rebounding with the mini trampoline, the sit-down rebounder, and an oscillating machine. I do not have a set routine; I have several mini trampolines in the most frequently used parts of my home and office. It's rare that I am on one for more than 5 minutes. I am always so busy on the telephone or running errands that I frequently rebound while talking to somebody if I feel the conversation is going to last more than a few minutes.

I usually spend about 10 minutes first thing in the morning and again last thing in the evening on my oscillator as I watch the news and check the weather. The one I use most often can go from 1 to 50 cycles per second, but I have found that it is difficult to carry on a conversation over the telephone when I am on a setting of more than 10 repetitions per second.

I have been using the mini trampoline and sit-down rebounder for 20 years, but have only added the oscillator in the past year. They used to sell from $10,000 to $20,000, which is way out of my price range. I am so thankful for my oscillator; I feel it has made a huge difference in my health and overall physical condition.

The oscillator was originally created for Russian astronauts. The technology has been used in the United States for over 20 years now by NASA and the U.S. Air Force in their pilot physical training programs. Prior to the introduction of this technology, the average pilot would black out at around 7 G's. Within 2–3 months of using the oscillator in their physical fitness program, they extended the limit up to 9 G's. This demonstrates the importance of the technology in our overall physical health. While the repetition of the rebounder adds stress to every cell of the body, stimulating its ability to excrete waste and take in nutrients, the oscillator stimulates each cell electrically, many times more rapidly than the rebounder can. My unit moves me back and forth, up and down from 1 to 50 times a second, as I choose. The company's research shows that 10 minutes on an oscillator is the equivalent of walking 4 miles. I have been using one for a little over a year now, and as of the end of 2011, I believe it to be true.

I am just now able to take it up to 40 cycles per second without some discomfort in my liver area. It took me 2–3 months to go beyond 10 cycles per second and an additional 3 months to go beyond 20. I will take it up to 50 within the next couple of months, I hope. I bought the machine about a year after being diagnosed with stage 4 liver cirrhosis. I was told to go home and get my affairs in order. The doctor said that the only treatment was a liver transplant, and I was too old to be a candidate. He made me determined to prove him wrong, and I have.

I had already made fantastic improvements before I bought my first oscillator, but using it along with rebounding, I can definitely see additional improvement. I feel sure that this is one of the things that have helped me in overcoming my liver problem.

Anything we can do to improve our cellular health and increase the flow of the lymph fluid is helpful. This is the primary reason that exercise is so important. Any long-term restriction in flow can cause some serious health issues.

One thing that really bothers me is that doctors actually cut lymph glands from people's bodies. I have had many friends endure this type of operation. It may have bought them a little time in their fight against cancer, but most of them lost the battle.

One cannot cleanse the body without understanding the lymph system and the critical part exercise plays in keeping the lymph fluid moving. All health starts with cleansing, detoxing, and ridding the body of pathogens and environmental toxins, followed by nutrition and exercise to strengthen the body.

Here are a few pieces of equipment and activities that can really make a difference in a person's life, and they are affordable (these are 2011 prices) and accessible to nearly everyone in the world:

A. Sodium Chlorite (MMS)—Oxidizes pathogens, carcinogens, and environmental toxins. At present, a 4-ounce bottle retails for $20 and lasts between 3 months and a year.

B. Diatomaceous Earth (DE)—this is 90 percent silica housed in a microscopic shell. A one-month supply costs between $30 and $50. A one-pound bag in bulk form, costs about $10 and lasts 2 months. Once DE releases its silica content into cells, the "empty shell" has a strong negative charge that attracts toxins (most toxins carry a positive charge) that are then "trapped" inside the shell until the DE is expelled from the body in stools. Once clean, the immune system is much more effective and efficient.

C. A mini trampoline—A good-quality one runs between $300 and $500. If you cannot afford that, try a jump rope from the dollar store. Aim for a combination of what you can afford and what you can do.

D. An oscillator—There are many on the market today, ranging in price from a few hundred to more than $20,000. The information I have read is that 10 minutes on one gives the equivalent of walking 4 miles, and I believe it. You can see a selection at www.A2ZhealthProducts.com.

E. Walking in the park—there are many parks with exercise trails (these have stops along the way where there are suggestions of exercises you can do) at no expense at all.

F. Chi machine—Helps move lymph fluid as well as stimulate the life force, our vital electric energy. This is not taught in the United States, but the Chinese have used it for thousands of years. The energy from the chakras creates our aura. We are energy beings, and our bodies, minds, and souls are all one and influenced by this energy.

G. Yoga—free classes are held at many community centers, senior centers, parks, and recreation centers. It is all about stretching, strengthening, and learning deep breathing techniques to allow more oxygen into the body, not about hard physical exercise. You can do it at your own pace.

My dad had a great sense of humor and had a joke for every situation. One of his more memorable stories was to help prepare me for getting old.

He said the hardest thing for him was the forgetfulness. He first noticed it whenever he would go to the bathroom; he was forgetting to shake it off before he zipped up. He always remembered soon after, as he felt something warm running down his leg for a couple of minutes afterward. Before long, he would forget to zip it up, and then shortly after that, he was forgetting to zip it down before going in the first place! "Old age is hell," he would say.

I like to look at the bright side of everything, but that did not get me excited about growing old. He painted such a bleak picture. The fact is, we are all getting older every day; it's inevitable, unless you and Dr. Kevorkian choose the alternative. I now believe we have other options, and I love feeling 20 years old.

No one can improve or even maintain good health without exercise. I can now walk much longer and faster than I could just 2 years ago, and I feel fantastic. I really want to encourage everyone to exercise in some way. Keep that lymph system moving and stay healthy.

Through exercise, pure water, nutrition, and internal body cleansing, we can have good health for free. We do not have to accept what is considered the norm. We can get back that clarity of thought and of mind, and that great feeling of youthfulness once again, without aches and pains. I love feeling youthful; I am really looking forward to the next 100 years, and I believe I will still feel 20 as I do today.

CHAPTER 13

Nutrition

Diets do not work, and everyone knows it. However, good nutrition does work, and it is easier than we think. It's more about what food we eat, the supplements we take, and what we don't need to eat, rather than how much we eat. Supplements are very important, as our food supply is mineral deficient and has been for many years. Minerals are the foundation of cellular life, our life, and our health. The only way to make sure we are assimilating all the needed bioavailable minerals is through proper digestion of supplements made from organically grown whole food sources. Once the body gets the nutrition it needs, it reduces cravings for more food, making it easy to maintain a healthy body and weight. "It is not what we eat, but what we assimilate that satisfies our hunger," states nutripath, Dr. Sal D'Onofrio.

Fat stores toxins that burden or overwhelm our immune system, making it very difficult to stay healthy. More people are becoming aware of the importance of a healthy lifestyle, but most of us feel we have to starve ourselves and deprive ourselves of the things we really want to eat. I eat what I want, when I want, and I feel better than I did when I was in my twenties.

There are two primary things that cause cravings that lead to overeating and obesity. The first we touched on above: the lack of minerals and other nutrients in what we eat, and the second is fungus.

Whenever I have had a serious health problem, I adjusted my diet to help me overcome the immediate health challenge, usually only for a short time. As soon as the crisis is over, I return to eating whatever and whenever I want to. However, there is more to the story.

When I fell back into my old eating habits and regained weight, my health issue would come back, or sometimes a new one would appear. Drs. Hitt and Humiston taught me about the harmful effects of *Candida*. Once I understood it and got it under control, both weight and health became simple to me.

1. I got rid of the fungus that controlled my brain chemistry and made me crave what *it* wanted to eat.

2. I cleansed and detoxed my body, getting rid of all the other pathogens and environmental pollutants that broke down my immune system.

3. I changed my diet to approximately 80 percent fresh fruits and vegetables that are nearly all alkaline, and 20 percent meat and foods that create acidity.

4. I limit my intake of food that is high in sugars and starches, as well as most grains and dairy. While addressing a health challenge, I do not eat them at all for 1–3 months.

5. Once I stop having cravings, I continue the diet and supplementing for 3–4 additional weeks before adding back anything I know is not good for me.

Life cannot come from death, so when we cook the life out of our food, we destroy most of its benefits. I also learned that root vegetables contain most of their nutrients close to the skin. The most nutrient-dense part of most fruits and vegetables that grow on trees or vines is in the center or core. This knowledge has helped me a great deal in understanding how to prepare what I eat.

Meeting Doug Widdifield and learning how to cook vegetables properly has made a big difference in my life and health. When I ate one of Doug Widdifield's meals, it blew me away. Of course, when I find something new to learn about health, I become obsessed. I began spending as much time as possible with Doug, learning all I could about waterless cookware, how to cook with it, and all the added benefits of using almost no water and very little heat. Now I not only get the maximum nutrient value from what I eat, but I can taste its true flavor, and it's very good. In fact, I can prepare a variety of vegetable dishes that are quite delicious.

I have used a pressure cooker for almost 50 years, because it made sense to me to use less water. Cooking vitamins and minerals in water pulls them out of the food and into the water, which is then poured down the drain. My earliest memory (before WWII was over) is of my mother and grandmother teaching me that; it has stuck with me all my life. But I vividly recall an incident from Christmas, 1944. My mother, grandmother, and two of her sisters were cooking Christmas dinner at our home using a large pressure cooker, and it exploded. It was as if a bomb went off in our house, and to me as a young child, it sounded like the war news that was always on the radio at the time. It was very scary to me, and it happened right in my home.

When I got married in 1960, one of our wedding presents was a pressure cooker. I asked my mom, "What were you thinking?" I could not imagine ever using it, as I had a subconscious fear of it. She explained how much more beneficial it was than conventional cooking. She also told me that the one that had blown up had had no pressure safety valve. Although I have 4 different sizes at my home right now, and I still use them from time to time, but I use waterless cookware more often.

With a pressure cooker, you cook under pressure at over 200°F, while with waterless cookware, you cook in a vacuum at a temperature ranging between 140 and 180°F.Some nutrients still cannot survive at those temperatures, but many more are unlocked for us to use.

Much of the nutrition in vegetables is located in the fiber, which causes a controversy between those who choose to eat raw food versus cooked. I had wondered about this for years: how could people have such vast differences of opinion on such an important matter? You would think that if our government really wanted to make a difference in our health, it would allocate money toward researching the matter.

Since December 2008, I have been learning more and more about how to cook to get the maximum flavor and nutrition from all foods. I improve my health, I save time, I get the maximum value for my money, and enjoy what I eat. I like win-win situations, so this is a very important part of understanding the benefits of nutrition for me.

I do eat raw vegetables as well and add some to my side dishes. I also start my day by juicing either fruits or vegetables, depending on what is in season. I have had a Vita Mix for at least 15 years, and it is the most used appliance in my home; I still use it nearly every day. I do not combine fruits and vegetables on the same morning, except that sometimes I juice watermelon several days in a row. However, I often mix a combination of fruits or a combination of vegetables, but when I juice melons, I don't mix anything with them. I have read that it is not a good idea to combine anything with melons; however, I do add supplements to all juices.

There is so much to learn about nutrition; it could evolve into a book itself. Getting nutrition in its best form is very important to understand. Getting nutrients from food is the best possible way. It will even have micronutrients we haven't begun to figure out yet.

I still struggle with eating organic, as the cost is so much higher than commercially grown crops; it is hard for me to justify the difference in price. If I were convinced that everything that claimed to be organic, truly was, it would be a much easier decision. Know the difference between "organic" and "certified organic." If it grows, it is organic in nature; but only certified is guaranteed to be without pesticides. There is just too much information suggesting that much of what is labeled as organic (and what we pay twice as much for) often really is not.

Just remember that "commercially grown" means "sprayed with poison." Soaking sprayed foods in 2 tablespoons of Clorox bleach (or my personal preference, 10 drops of Sodium Chlorite (MMS)), mixed in a gallon of water, will remove some poisons, then rinse and cook, but many poisons are locked in fiber of the crop and not released until heat is applied.

I often go to Whole Foods and other similar health food stores looking for organic vegetables that are reasonably priced. If any are priced within 20–30 percent of commercially grown, I buy. At 50 to 100 percent greater, I do not. That is just my yardstick, and I am not suggesting anyone else use it. Since I don't know anyone healthier than I am for my age (or any age, for that matter), or anyone who feels better than I do, my policy seems to have worked well for me. Keep in mind that I am nearly always on some form of cleanse. That may be why I continue to thrive on a large percentage of commercially grown foods. If I could afford to buy everything organic, I probably would. I feel sure that you would be better off doing so if money is no object.

By eliminating (or I should say, dramatically reducing) the amount of pathogens in my body, and taking the most nutrient-dense supplements I know of (spirulina, wheatgrass, hemp and pea protein, rice bran, and rice solubles), I have no craving for the more harmful foods. There may be hundreds, if not thousands, of other trace nutrients science has not yet discovered that our body needs or can use. Most vitamins and minerals that are not from a whole food source are worthless anyway, because the body cannot assimilate them, and they do not have all the micronutrients that allow them to work synergistically. Whole foods are so nutrient dense that there is a good chance many of the undiscovered nutrients are also in them, and our bodies can use them now. I also noticed that I can control my tinnitus by increasing green food nutrients and backing off high-fat and high-sugar foods. Staying away from carbs, fats, and sugars is easy when you have no cravings.

Our bodies need at least 100 nutrients every day, according to what I read and science knows of today. We also need 60 minerals, 16 vitamins, 8 essential amino acids, and 3 essential fatty acids every day, plus more. A few new ones have been discovered in recent years. I think Dr. Wallach has done a great service for humankind and believe he has done a fantastic job of making people aware of the body's need for not just any minerals, but those derived from plant sources, which are 100 percent bioavailable at the cellular level.

In his tape from about 1996, Dr. Wallach points out that "Dead Doctors Don't Lie," and that food manufacturers add 40 minerals to dog food but only 10 to baby food. I don't know whether you've had the same experience I did, but my kids were sick more often than my dogs. Does it make sense that our animal's food is better than ours, and that they receive better nutritional advice from a veterinarian than we do from a medical doctor? It makes you wonder what the life expectancy of a veterinarian is compared to that of a medical doctor. The last statistic I saw for a medical doctor was only 58 years, while the average person in the United States was 72 years old. Today our average age is up to 78, but the AMA will not release updated statistics for their membership. This leads me to believe it is, at least in part, from the lack of nutritional education required in conventional medicine.

By reducing fungal load, we can reduce the desire to overeat. Sodium Chlorite (MMS), a very affordable water purification product, can be very effective in reducing all forms of pathogens. Once the viral and fungal load is reduced and the body's need for minerals is balanced, we gradually gravitate to a normal healthy body weight without diet, and health will improve dramatically. Health and weight control can be just that simple, since the body naturally surrounds many toxins with fat for its own survival.

Lose weight + lose toxins = health, a simple formula to improve health. When we get pathogens and environmental toxins out of our bodies and support our immune systems with balanced nutrition, the body will heal itself.

Everyone has an opinion on nutrition and there are valid points to support different lines of reasoning. I will share some of these with you in the hope that you will develop your own beliefs and find what works for you. I encourage you to keep looking for the right person or products that can change your life and your health. Through prayer, a positive mental attitude, and perseverance, the answers will come to you.

It is all about internal balance in what we eat, drink, and breathe. I have heard many doctors state that they will no longer take a patient who will not quit smoking, as there is little hope in helping anyone who won't help themselves.

I am thankful that my taste has adapted toward eating vegetables, since they are very healthy. I also like to eat a lot of greens and salads. In my younger years, I lived on meat and potatoes, pasta and bread, sandwiches, a lot of dairy products, milk shakes, and dessert. I drank carbonated beverages and canned juices—just about anything but water.

Now I drink mostly water, freshly juiced fruit, or vegetable juice. My day usually starts with fruit juice mixed with a little vegetable protein, vitamin C, diatomaceous earth, stabilized rice bran, rice solubles, spirulina, and wheatgrass. I also supplement with a few other things like Optimum D-Tox, a natural whole food that helps cleanse the insides and has other health benefits. I take natural-state iodine and magnesium/calcium for bone support and balanced Minerals of Life, in which most of us are deficient.

About noon, if I am at home, I eat mostly vegetables and salads with a little chicken, fish or turkey for added protein, or a little jack or pepper jack cheese. I still eat a hamburger every week or two and have a milkshake once or twice a month. However, while overcoming some of my more serious health challenges, I went for several years without cheating much.

For lunch on the run, I eat whatever is convenient, since I am out taking care of business, at a health trade show, or having lunch with a doctor or someone in the health field. This is usually my largest meal, and it nearly always includes meat in some form.

My nighttime meal is often mostly vegetables I cook myself in waterless cookware, and I often add some goat cheese to it just before I take it out of the pan, I often have salad with it. Probably 3 times a week, I add a small piece of fish or chicken.

Now I feel comfortable eating just about anything I want, when I want. But I now recognize the first sign of a craving as a sign that fungus is coming back. The cravings quickly go away if I take Sodium Chlorite (MMS) for 4–6 weeks and a bottle or two of Molecula Silver. If the cravings are not gone in 6 weeks, I use a jar of Yeast Control; so far, it has worked very well.

Chi is the principle used by acupuncture practitioners throughout the world. Some people can see this energy or aura, and there are cameras that can photograph it now. There are many reasons we could have energy blockages in our chi that can have negative effects on our health. If this is completely new to you and you find it hard to comprehend why we're not taught this, I understand; but I assure you, it is true. 20 years ago, I found it hard to believe this energy existed if everyone didn't know about it. Now I realize it is so important to health, and still only a small percentage of Americans know about it. After attending dozens of workshops and lectures on magnetic energy, radionics, acupuncture, and many others on related energy fields, I am convinced that our chakras generate energy and affect the body's health.

The body is electrical. We have two electrical systems; they are both dependent on minerals to maintain communication. We are more familiar with the electrical nervous system, but there is one more. This energy field, which is little known in the United States, is referred to the life force (more commonly known as *chi* in Chinese medicine). Its existence has been proven with Kirlian photography. This energy field creates our aura. Now there are scientific instruments that can measure chi. It allows every cell to understand the body's needs and to participate in fulfilling them. Healthy cells make a healthy body, and inner-cellular communication requires minerals. However, minerals are not a silver bullet that will cure all diseases by themselves. They are just one of the body's requirements for balancing and maintaining our health.

1. We must understand how to balance our body's needs to allow the immune system to keep us healthy. Just a little understanding of nutrition can make a difference: the 22 amino acids make approximately 50,000 combinations of cellular interactions necessary to function and stay healthy. They come from protein foods like grains, sprouts, legumes, beans, and flesh foods like meat that is not overcooked, and natural, unprocessed fat and oil. Bee pollen is also a very good source of all 22 amino acids.

2. Vitamins and minerals are best from a natural whole food source. Supplement with spirulina, wheatgrass, stabilized rice bran, and all-natural iodine, as there is so little of it in what we eat. When we have a health challenge that might be related to a vitamin or mineral shortage, we often need additional supplementation.

3. Enzymes are critical for all cellular repairs. Our body naturally makes an adequate amount until we are about 30 years old; after that, we are largely dependent on fresh fruits , vegetables and supplements. There are 2,000–3,000 of them; only some are needed for digestion, which is just a small part of their function. Taking more vitamins than the body has enzymes to utilize can create another health problem in itself, as an overdose of vitamins without the balance of other nutrients can be toxic.

4. I am not claiming to be an expert in any of this; I am simply passing on what I have learned, along with nutrition guidelines that have worked for me. I have met many doctors who believe the same as I do and who practice the same principles of self-healing through balancing the body's needs.

CHAPTER 14

Water

Water is essential to life and health. Our bodies are 70–80 percent water. The number given differs depending on the source of the information, but they all agree that every drop of our water is replaced often. But what does "often" mean? I have read it can be as often as every 2 weeks. This is, of course, impossible, because as I would need to drink more than 2 gallons of water a day at my body weight. No matter how often the replacement really is, it is the fastest way to rid our bodies of waste, so it's logical to me that the first thing we should do is drink a lot of pure water.

I first started learning about water around 1995 when I found out about this replacement process. I realized that I needed to learn a lot more.

Tom Brokaw did a segment about water in January 1997 on NBC News. I started documenting what I learned with several startling facts from this broadcast:

1. More than 100 people died from contaminated drinking water in a city in the Midwest.

2. In the 3 previous years, more than 10,000,000 people were told to boil their drinking water because municipal water systems were inadequate in the United States.

3. 1 out of every 15 households drank bottled water.

4. Lead in old plumbing caused many health problems.

Dr. Joseph M. Price stated, "Chlorine is the biggest killer and crippler of modern time. While it prevented epidemics of one disease, it is creating another." He, along with many other doctors, believes that many of our nation's health problems come from chlorine. It is a poison!

This broadcast had such a profound impact on me that I became a water fanatic. I was sure there would be many more national news stories following up on this, but in all the news I have watched I have not seen anything with as much real impact. It brought back to mind that all life, as we know it, is dependent on water. Pure water (not any old tap water) is a necessity for a healthy life.

(The above was taken from my notes from 1997. I wish I could verify the facts as they are today before I finish my book, but I have been working on writing it for so many years now that I just don't want to take the time. I ask that any reader who would like to comment on any subject in my book to please direct comments to INFO@YourHealthisYourChoice.org.)

On my *Health Talk Radio* show, I had recommended that everybody read the book, *Your Body's Many Cries for Water*, by Dr. Batmanghelidj, MD.

He has an incredible story. He was a wealthy Iranian doctor living in Tehran when Khomeini came to power. Every one of means was arrested, sentenced to death, and their property confiscated. Thousands were held in a prison designed to hold 600. Every day the guards would take 30 or 40 men outside and shoot them. The number largely depended on how many graves the guards felt like digging that day. All this was obviously very stressful to the minds and bodies of the inmates. The food was of poor quality, and sickness and disease ran rampant.

Dr. Batmanghelidj was in charge of taking care of the sick. There was absolutely no medicine of any kind available. No matter what a patient's problem was, all he could do was give them water. He was so inspired by its results in many types of diseases that he started documenting the miraculous cures. This made such an impact on the prison officials that they granted him a pardon and offered to release him. He begged to be allowed to stay and finish his research.

In his book he says that in the United States alone, 1,000,000 people are killed and $700 billion is wasted annually treating thirst-related illnesses with drugs. He also states that most pain is a sign of dehydration. Dr. Batmanghelidj has done great work, and all of us here in the United States can learn from him. I feel we all owe him our gratitude. In my opinion, he must have been blessed having good pure water; otherwise he surely would not have had these results.

After reading his book and understanding the importance of water better, I opened my own water store to ensure that my family, friends, and I were getting the purest possible water. I learned to test water myself to maintain the best quality. This experience led me to start *Health Talk Radio* on KLAV in Las Vegas so I could share the important things I learned about water and health.

(Seawater, with its natural mineral balance, seems to be the basis of all life; it has the same mineral content as our blood. We cannot drink it, because the salinity is too high. But knowing that natural sea salt has all the minerals in the correct proportion helps me understand how some life forms could have evolved from the sea.)

Once I knew that the body's water content ranged between 70 and 80 percent, it made sense to me to drink a lot of pure water. This is one of the most important ways to help our bodies regain and maintain health. My water store sparked a renewed interest in learning all I could about water. I thought I completely understood water and its many benefits, but by the year 2000, I got bored and shut down my store. Now I realize there is much more to understand about water's benefits than I thought ten years ago.

In 2011, I was introduced to Double Helix Water. I put 5 drops in a quart of water filtered by reverse osmosis just before I went to bed. I slept for 8 straight hours without waking up for anything; this is very rare for me. The few times it did, I wrote it down upon waking so I wouldn't forget what I felt made it possible. Some things that have helped worked for a few days to a few weeks but did not offer lasting benefits. Sleep is a very important part of staying healthy.

When I woke up on January 21, 2011, I was also experiencing sexual feelings for the first time in 20 years. Even though I overcame prostate cancer back then, I never got back a natural physical desire for sex. A few things have helped (see Chapter 6), but none of them had a lasting benefit. Obviously, it is too soon to tell if the helix water will, but I feel it is important to remember what happened that morning.

My health would improve and symptoms would go away so subtly that I did not realize it until they came back. Sometimes they reappeared in weeks or even a year or more, but because I had not written it down, I was not able to recall what I had done or taken that may have helped the first time.

This is why I encourage everyone to keep a health log, like a diary. Follow the steps outlined in Chapter 11. I have not always been as diligent as I should be about this, but have found it to be one of the most important things I have done, as it has been a big part of my education in reversing my health issues.

General health is simple, it's true; but once I move beyond a major disease issue, I become a fanatic who wants to fine-tune my health in an effort to become as perfect as possible. I truly feel we have the potential to live for hundreds of years and remain feeling 20 years old. I believe the FDA is suppressing much of today's technology because of the obvious collusion with the pharmaceutical companies. With much of the research by independent individuals as well as scientists and doctors, the truth is not adequately disseminated.

I can see why many medical doctors find a specialty they want to focus on, since some aspects of health are very complicated. I still believe that only the body can heal itself when given the opportunity. However, if it were not for doctors like David L. Gann and Shui-yin Lo doing the research they have, this remarkable water would not have been discovered. They not only have the education to develop it, but the ability to explain it to the average person like myself in a way that we can understand it and to encourage us to try it.

After taking the Double Helix Water the first night, I felt hypnotized when I woke up and realized I had slept for 8 straight hours and in a state of relaxation I could not ever recall before. I just laid there enjoying the incredible feeling for about a half an hour, and then I wrote it down, as I did not want to ever forget the experience.

I drank 6 more ounces that morning and continued throughout the day. I was under a lot of stress with many things that would normally exhaust me. Being in touch with how stress affects my body, I was amazed at how well I was able to deal with it. I did not feel the tension that usually wears me out under such abnormally stressful periods. The feeling of relaxation stayed with me throughout the day. If you have ever experienced the benefits of an adaptogen, you may be able to relate, but most will not be able to understand what I am trying to explain until they have experienced it.

The next day I drank another 6 ounces just before bed. I was able to finish my prayer and did not forget to thank God for all my blessings. Just before lights out, as the relaxation once again came over me, I specifically thanked him for the water and my friend Tracy Tucker for introducing me to it. I think I did wake up once that night, but enjoying the feeling of total relaxation, I was out like a light again. I was aware of several dreams that night, but was not aware of any the night before. Even though I could not recollect what I was dreaming about, I do remember the circumstances, and they were all tranquil.

The next morning I also woke in complete relaxation. As soon as I finished writing that morning, I made a gallon of water for my daughter, her husband, and my grandson, who live next door. They all had some health issues that need to be addressed. I couldn't seem to get them to stay on Sodium Chlorite (MMS) long enough to make a difference, but they all drank a lot of water.

On January 24, I was asleep in about 10 minutes, but did not notice the relaxing, hypnotic type of feeling I had had the previous 2 nights; I believed the benefits of the water were diminishing. I woke up once to go to the bathroom, as I had drunk a lot of water, but this time I fell asleep again, feeling relaxed. On my 4th night, it took me about 20 minutes to get to sleep. I did not feel the relaxation that I had the first 2 nights, but I slept well through the night and woke up relaxed.

My friend Tracy told me that she mixed a bottle of the water and went grocery shopping. She sat down at a table there, drank 6 ounces of water, and started to read a book. In 10 minutes, she fell asleep. She and I must have needed whatever is in it more than most. I gave this water to my children, who are all in their forties, and they did not experience what we did. They all have their own health problems, and not one of them noticed anything at all. I was not sure if the water really detoxed, as I may not have been nearly as toxic as they. Three of them told me they felt it kept them awake. I know what they eat, and none have ever been diligent with cleanses.

By May 2011, I had been drinking this water for 4 months. I continued to sleep 6 to 8 hours a night and still felt 20 years old, but when you already feel as good as I do, it is very difficult to feel better—so it is increasingly difficult to evaluate new products. I still had half of my first bottle, so it was not as expensive as I thought it might be; at that rate it would end up costing no more than $25 a month. I decided to continue to use it and recommend it to others, because I was handling the stress of life with far less noticeable tension than usual. Before I started drinking it, I was in denial of stress. I just didn't realize how much stress affected me. After experiencing the difference in relaxation, I have no doubt that trying to run a business and working over 100 hours a week put me under a lot of stress over the past few years.

Please remember that balanced minerals, pure water, the sun's life-giving energy, the earth's magnetic energy and fresh air are essential to life and health. They are affordable and will play a big part in making *Your Health Your Choice*. Only you can do this for yourself.

CHAPTER 15

Environment

No bugs, no life. I don't know if you are old enough to remember when someone washed your windshield every time you bought gas. About the time self-serve gas stations started, there was a big drive to get rid of bugs without using DDT, which we were told back in the 1950s was detrimental to the environment. I do not know what they used to replace DDT, but it seems it has done a very good job in most parts of the country. I just wonder if the new chemicals could possibly have been more harmful than the DDT.

In 1951, my family moved from Illinois to Nevada. We had made several trips back and forth over the following few years, at least one each summer. My dad was rarely satisfied with the window-washing job the service station attendants did. If he wasn't, it was my job to do it again. I remember when there were so many bugs on our windows that after 10 or15 minutes, my dad would have to finish my job. Now it is rare if I hit a bug of any size, much less a rabbit.

While driving from Charleston, South Carolina, to Las Vegas in May 2000, I reminisced about my many trips between Illinois and Nevada over the past 50 years. On every trip, I recall seeing hundreds of rabbits, if not thousands, along with quite a few foxes, coyotes, and many skunks. I recall two occasions when the rabbits were so thick we were hitting 10–20 of them per mile. Many times, they went in every direction—even right into the side of our car. It was impossible to miss them, even slowing down to 25 or 30 miles an hour. It was like driving through a cloud of locusts. Both times this was at night, once in Nevada and the other in Wyoming. Aside from the few rabbits I see running free near my house, I recall thinking, I have not seen rabbits or even road kill on a highway in the last couple of years, and I drive a lot.

Through some states, it used to be normal to see deer, opossum, badgers, raccoons, a weasel now and then, and always quite a number of snakes that had been hit along the road. Yet on the trip in 2000, I never needed to wash my windows or even scrape a bug off the windshield until I reached Arizona and finally hit my first! I did not see a rabbit or any other living animal, again, not even road kill.

On another trip, in 2001, I heard a doctor on the radio in Florida talking about health. He claimed the average oxygen content of our air is now 16 percent. I found this hard to believe, because when I started volunteering for the fire department in 1955, we were taught that the oxygen content was 21 percent. In 1961, when I got out of the Marine Corps and started working as a full-time firefighter, they were still teaching us the same number. They continued to teach it until I retired in 1991, and to my knowledge that has not changed.

It is hard to imagine that we could lose 5 percent of our oxygen in just over 40 years. That 5 percent reduction equals approximately a 25 percent loss of the oxygen in our atmosphere over a 40-year period—that is beyond imagination. The doctor on the radio in 2001 was the first one I heard mention that 16 percent. By now, 10 years later, I have heard many other doctors lecturing at health trade shows make similar statements. Our oxygen level has been, and continues to be, depleted. I have not heard one person explain the cause adequately or offer any solution. For our planet to continue to sustain life, one would think this is something we should be aware of so we can start making the corrections needed.

The earth's atmosphere contained 38 percent oxygen as recently as the mid-19th century. The Industrial Revolution in the 1880s brought the burning of fossil fuels, industrial pollution, and eventually, car exhaust. By the 1950s, the percentage of oxygen in our atmosphere had dropped to 21 percent. Although 21 percent is still normally quoted as our current level, recent tests indicate that the oxygen level may now be at only 19 percent on average. In the heart of many large industrial cities, the percent of oxygen may test as low as 16 percent.

(Note: The above information I found in my notes several times from different lectures I attended over the past 20 years. I have not taken the time to research just what the latest facts are at this time. If you feel this is not accurate information and take the time to research it, I would like to see your findings. Please send an e-mail to me at INFO@YourHealthisYourChoice.org.)

It is scary to see these major changes in our environment within my own lifetime. This has heightened my awareness of the toxic environment we now live in and helps me better understand the need to cleanse and detoxify my organs in my effort to maintain my personal health. We all need to do this.

I recall reading an article in the '60s that the largest deer herd in the United States was in Pennsylvania. I drove through that state at night a few years ago and did not see one deer, dead or alive. The fencing along the freeway is a good deterrent, but I know deer can get through the fences, as I have seen them jump much higher ones with no problem at all. I did not see a rabbit or fox or any other living thing either, nor did I get a bug on my windshield.

The Fish and Game Department told me that there are more deer in Nevada now than ever in the state's history. I cannot prove whether this is true or not, but I have not seen many when I've gone camping. I like to take photos of wildlife now, as I no longer hunt; however, I see only about 5 percent of the deer I once saw. It is as rare to see any other wildlife along the highway as other states I've mentioned. I drive several thousands of miles through Nevada alone; some areas range in excess of 50 miles between gas stations. In the past few years, I have only seen wildlife in the northwestern states, but still nowhere near the numbers I used to.

I have lived on a half an acre 4 miles from McCarran Airport near Las Vegas for 30 years. The town has grown for miles past my once-rural home, and yet I have seen more coyotes in my yard in the past few years than anyplace else in the United States except Idaho. Fortunately, coyotes are quite amazing in their ability to adapt to changing conditions and encroachment by increased population. It seems like it was only a few years ago that I was hunting cottontail and quail here. Just a few miles away, we had a dude ranch until 1983 where we could ride horses in nearly every direction for miles without running across a neighbor with a fence, and only a few paved roads would restrict our travel.

At this time in Las Vegas, it is difficult to find vacant land that you could ride a horse on, much less the 70 horses we had and the 6 teams for our hay wagons. Fortunately, I can still see some of the remnants of the past able to survive; I continue to see rabbits, quail, and coyotes around my home at least once or twice a week.

This is just an illustration of the changes in our environment that I have seen in my lifetime. It has raised my awareness and understanding that my grandchildren and great-grandchildren will have far worse challenges than we have faced over the past 70 years. The air and water pollution in the valley, along with the lack of water, is taking a toll on our quality of life. I personally believe that these toxic environmental problems directly relate to the increase in diseases we are experiencing that previous generations never had to deal with.

Water quality and the amount of increase use of chlorine nationwide:

In the early 1950s, I would spend days at Lake Mead, Nevada. The water was so clean and clear; it felt as though I could see 100 feet or more down into the lake. I thought nothing of drinking right out of it and never got so much as a stomach ache. In the 1960s, I noticed a decline in the depth I could see into the water; by the 1970s, I would no longer consider drinking from Lake Mead after a serious bout with diarrhea that lasted several days that I believe came from drinking out of the lake.

In 2011, I find it difficult to see 3–4 feet into the water; and without the use of ozone and/or chlorine to purify it, drinking that water may be fatal today. However, I have heard several kinds of doctors state that the increased use of chlorine for maintaining safe drinking water directly correlates with the increases in many diseases that either did not exist 30 years ago or were of little consequence.

After personally using Sodium Chlorite (MMS) for nearly 5 years, I have noticed many health benefits. I have heard thousands success stories from people around the world. I believe it is the most important health discovery of my lifetime. Sodium Chlorite (MMS) is not only the best choice for water purification, it can clean the blood, the mind, and the circulatory system. Its oxidation has lowered my weight and blood pressure and given me clarity of thought I have not had since I was in my twenties.

I took a science class at community college in 1971 or '72 to complete my degree in fire science and a second degree in business administration. I chose environmental science, since I thought it would be the easiest. I went into it with little respect for tree huggers, but by the time I finished, I was one of them. This class changed my life more than any other. I now feel that a student should not be able to graduate from high school without at least one semester in environmental science.

I have become much more environmentally aware in recent years. If we are killing off all the bugs, wildlife, and the creatures of the sea, what are we doing to ourselves?

I really cannot state often enough that our health really is our choice. It is imperative that we understand the simplicity of eliminating, or at least reducing, the pathogens and environmental toxins that break down our immune system so our bodies can heal themselves. This truly is health made simple, and it is affordable to the poorest people in the world. Sodium Chlorite (MMS) is just one of a number of things that Jim Humble has discovered through his research that has the potential to change the world.

The human cost is overwhelming; the economic cost also is one of the most devastating problems our nation faces. The costs of treating these conditions are tremendous without even taking into consideration the cost of the many secondary health problems they cause; this alone was estimated to be $277 billion in 2003. These conditions also reduce productivity at the workplace, as ill employees and their caregivers are often forced either to miss work or work at a reduced capacity. The impact of this loss in productivity and time lost at work is reported to be in the billions of dollars each year.

The number of cases in the United States is listed below, along with its percentage of the population, based on the prevalence of the 7 more common chronic diseases. It would be interesting to know how much more loss in productivity is due to injury, because back injury and pain are very high on the list of causes of time lost at work as well. This, again, is simple and inexpensive to address and would save employers not only millions to billions in lost time and productivity, but it would also save our most valuable assets, our citizens, pain and suffering.

Pulmonary Conditions: 49,206,000 (17.4 percent)
Hypertension: 36,761,000 (13.0 percent)
Mental Disorders: 30,338,000 (10.7 percent)
Heart Disease: 19,145,000 (6.8 percent)
Diabetes: 13,729,000 (4.9 percent)
Cancers: 10,555,000 (3.7 percent)
Stroke: 2,425,000 (0.9 percent)

The above is considered as percentages of the non-institutionalized population (those not in some form of forced confinement). The number of treated cases is based on patient self-reported data from 2003 Military Entrance Processing Stations (MEPS). This information is not a fair estimate, since it does not include untreated and undiagnosed cases.

I estimate that ninety percent of these health issues can be corrected with the use of Sodium Chlorite (MMS), ozone, and magnetic energy, based on what I have been able to do for myself.

I feel I have been 100 percent successful in reversing all of my health problems and many of my aging processes.

The younger population has not had the benefit of seeing for themselves the rapid decline in the quality of our water and air. I am afraid many won't realize what the future holds for them until it is too late to change our world. My generation is currently controlling our country; our congressmen and senators may have allowed our environment to regress too far for us to make a difference for our grandchildren.

We may have killed Planet Earth already; it just hasn't rolled over and died yet. It is conceivable that, because of humanity's greed and complacency in America's decadent lifestyle, we have been selling our land and giving our job market to foreign interests that have far less understanding of the environment's importance.

Because our elected leaders have chosen to do what is best to keep them in office, they have created a nightmare of laws and tax burdens. These have forced many of our most important industries, along with their technology, to outsource to other countries, leaving us without jobs, or even a base of skilled personnel capable of competing in our global market.

I now realize that there are many other things that are vital to supporting our way of life that have been outsourced to China. It seems that China now controls our destiny, since it controls such a large part of our debt as well as our former manufacturing capability. What do the Chinese think about the world's environment, human rights, or our way of life?

Our government's excuse is that we needed the strict laws to protect our environment. It seems to be a catch-22, since the laws simply add to the bureaucracy and have not accomplished much except to reduce our employment base. Every day there are more and more laws being passed restricting our constitutional freedoms?

I feel that the information in my book can help everyone by giving readers food for thought to find what will work for them if they are willing to accept responsibility for their own health and to have the desire and determination to improve their life.

CHAPTER 16

Teeth

By 2001, I had been having some problems with my teeth. I had an infection in my lower left molar and a cavity that needed to be filled. I also had to replace an upper right molar that had been extracted due to infection and breakage from a previous root canal. I needed a partial since I had been missing two teeth in my lower left jaw. One more was pulled in October, 2001; I had an infection that lasted for several months.

This was, of course, before I ran across Sodium Chlorite (MMS). I had gum pain in an area where I had had an extraction; as I mentioned earlier, my tooth issues may have been responsible for my heart attack and the sinus and ear infections that plagued me for several weeks at the time.

I had an abscessed tooth, but did not realize it until I bit down on something that caused a terrible pain in the right side of my month. I went to the dentist the next morning, but the X-rays only showed a long-term, low-grade infection in a left lower tooth, nothing in the right side.

I had been very successful in getting rid of small infections in my fingers using the negative side of small neodymium magnets. I was sure this would work on my tooth, so I slept with one taped to my lower jaw for about a month.

In late October, 2001, I bit down on something that caused such severe pain it felt like the roots of all my teeth had been exposed at once. The glands in my throat swelled up and throbbed; my eye, temple, and ear felt as though I was being hit with a two-by-four with every heartbeat. Tears flowed and my nose ran; it was as though all the pain was trying to exit through the top of my head. The strangest thing of all was that my lips became instantly chapped.

The next morning I went back to Dr. Oehlem for more X-rays, expecting to find that the infection had moved from the left side and had maybe settled in the right, adding to the severity of the pain. There was no noticeable change, and he could not identify the source of the pain. He assured me that whatever the problem was, it was not tooth related.

It was obvious that I had an infection in the right side of my head, as it was very swollen. The doctor gave me pain pills and antibiotics. The pain pills were of no value at all, and I soon found that walking was the only thing that gave me relief. If I sat down for 30 minutes or lay down for 20, the pain once again became unbearable.

I got another prescription for pain the same evening, but it did not help. Even doubling the amount did not help; I became nauseated and threw up a couple of times Monday night. I could only sleep about 20 minutes at a time and would wake up in such pain that I would have to get up and walk 5–10 minutes before lying down again.

Tuesday morning I went to urgent care to see a medical doctor, thinking it may be more than a toothache. He gave me a shot of antibiotics and one for pain. They both offered some relief. He prescribed more powerful antibiotics and pain pills than the dentist had and ordered a CAT scan, as he had no other idea what to look for. By that evening on the new pain medication, I was so nauseated I threw up about every 2 hours. I could only lie down for about 10 minutes, and it would take me 20–30 minutes to walk off the pain. I couldn't even sit for more than 10 minutes at a time.

The next morning, I went back to urgent care, but Dr. Wingard was off that day. Things seemed to be getting worse, and I felt I could not stand another night like the last one, so I went to the emergency room of a nearby hospital and checked in. They ran several tests, gave me a shot, and sent me home. I don't even remember getting home, but I woke up in bed 12 hours later and feeling pretty good for the first time in several days.

This is one time in my life I was very thankful for good drugs. I had become quite cynical about the service and knowledge of most medical doctors and medications. I have no idea what that doctor gave me, but it must have been some form of narcotic; it worked incredibly well. I definitely wanted more. Nothing else had worked, and it made me realize that I should be sympathetic to those who are addicted to drugs, because I could not have stood the pain any longer.

Thursday morning after getting up and moving around, a little pain returned. When I sat down for about 15 minutes, I was overwhelmed. I was able to walk it off to a tolerable level in about 30 minutes. I then tried to have breakfast, but the pain intensified when I tried to chew and swallow. I called my friend, Dr. Bonlie.

He assured me that it was not possible for magnets to push the infection to the right side of my head. His best guess was that the parotid gland was infected or blocked somehow. He thought that the motion of walking forced the lymph system to drain all areas of the body and to shrink the swelling, thus reducing the pain. This made sense to me, and I felt better knowing that the magnets hadn't added to the problem and why it helped to walk.

Because of my success in turning around all my health problems, I had not needed to see a doctor in nearly 5 years. I had become so arrogant that I had started telling people I did not expect to have another sick day as long as I was alive. I still expect to live to be at least 150 and remain productive with a great quality of life, but I now have a profound respect for medical doctors and some dentists. Dr. Bonlie remains at the top of my list.

The Rose de Lima Hospital emergency room doctor, Dr. Michael Kramer, had made an appointment with an eye, ear, nose, and throat specialist, Dr. David Martin, for me that afternoon. The specialist took more x-rays, additional tests, and gave me more prescriptions plus another shot. I went home and slept for another twelve hours, feeling nothing. He agreed with Dr. Bonlie about the parotid gland and scheduled me for an ultrasound on Wednesday.

In just 5 days, I saw 7 doctors, 3 of whom put me to sleep 3 days in a row. Without their help, I might have killed myself, as the pain was so unbearable. In the middle of the night, I would find myself banging my head against the wall trying to knock myself out before I finally broke down and went to the emergency room. This is just to give you an idea of my state of mind, since I had had bad experiences with doctors and hospitals. That is how badly I didn't want to go to the hospital and deal with the average MD.(One good thing is that I lost 10 pounds in 10 days; I always try to look at the bright side. If I had to go through this to lose weight, I would much prefer to die a young, fat man.)

I had been on antibiotics for 15 days when I went back to Dr. Olenderon on November 6. She opened up the tooth, let it drain some more, and put a new temporary filling in. It was already becoming a minor problem, as there was still some pain flaring up. The tooth finally broke and had to be pulled; with more antibiotics and a couple of more weeks to heal, the problem finally resolved. The pain and suffering were unbearable at times, all because of a dentist who could not read an X-ray, and my insurance paid thousands of dollars because of his incompetence.

I feel so bad for the millions of people without insurance. I really might have killed myself if the emergency room doctor had not put me to sleep when he had. I don't know whether socialized medicine could resolve the problem, but I do believe that at least expanded emergency room services should be available to everyone. At this time, only services for life-threatening situations are available in emergency rooms. Most doctors would not have found my circumstances life threatening; but I could not stand the pain and might have continued banging my head against the wall until I killed myself, caused permanent brain damage, or became unconscious.

This experience made me realize that even with cleansing, detoxing, nutrition, exercise, and building a strong immune system, it will not compensate for gradual tooth decay that could lead to infection, which overwhelms the immune system. It can make a big difference in the rest of your health and longevity.

As of January 2011, I feel certain I would not have lost any of my teeth if I had been brushing and flossing with Sodium Chlorite (MMS) 10 years ago (I have done so for 5 years now). All my gum disease is gone; I have no plaque on my teeth, and it has been 6 years since my teeth were cleaned. Sodium Chlorite (MMS) oxidizes the plaque from teeth, and I believe it does the same in the circulatory system. My blood pressure had run high for years; I had several doctors recommend medication for that and for diabetes, but I always refused. I have not had one doctor recommend that since I started using Sodium Chlorite (MMS). I would be very surprised if I ever get another tooth infection for the rest of my life. I have already noted that I believe my tooth problems contributed a great deal to my heart problems along with other health issues.

While hosting my *Health Talk Radio* show, around 1999 I was fortunate enough to interview Hal Huggins, DDS, who wrote *It's All in Your Head.* He believes that most health problems can be addressed with proper dental care. I was very impressed with Dr. Huggins then, and by now I have probably met more than 20 dentists who have trained under him. They all agree that eliminating mercury from fillings is one of the most important things a person can do to improve overall health.

I have spoken with hundreds of people who have had their mercury fillings removed and nearly all have reported tremendous improvement. I suggest that if you are having a health problem that is not responding as you feel it should, you may want to do the same and see if it helps.

Many dentists follow Dr. Huggins' methods, but if he did not supervise their training, I might not trust them to do the extraction properly. Proper safety measures include the use of dams to prevent saliva from running down the throat, and breathing the fumes as they must be exhausted while drilling, lest they cause further contamination and further health issues.

By March 2002, I had tried twice in 2 weeks to see Dr. Ashmend, who had been my dentist for nearly 40 years. He had been trying to retire for about a year, so he rescheduled me with Dr. Oehlem to fill a cavity I had developed between teeth. He had talked me into my first extraction in October 2001, causing all of my health problems. I had waited too long. A tooth had decayed to the point it could not be filled without getting into the root. It would need a root canal, which would weaken it too much to support a partial. I still had an infection near this tooth. It really upsets me that I knew what to do and how to get rid of it, yet did not take the time to do it. I guess because it was not painful at the time, I never thought about treating the infected area. My focus was more on my heart, and I didn't really understand the relationship between my teeth and my heart at that time. The anxiety of going to the dentist exacerbated discomfort in my heart, and I was now becoming more certain that my teeth were more directly related to my heart than I had previously thought.

Chinese medicine charts the chakras and meridians. Chakras provide energy to the meridians, which then provide energy to the organs. A meridian is best described as an electrical loop that passes through the mouth and 2 or 3 teeth. When the teeth are damaged, pulled, or infected, the electrical flow is blocked and this can affect an organ associated with that meridian. It can cause stress on an organ or, as in my case, a heart attack. This is my opinion based on my last 10 years of exploring all forms of healing available.

Even though I have learned a great deal more by now, I still believe this to be true. A friend recently pointed out to me that all health problems can be identified in the meridians long before they show up as diagnosable.

Many people do not believe in or don't understand the meridians and their effects on the body. I know it has taken me a long time to understand and accept their existence. I am a real believer now, since no one has offered any other logical explanation that would explain my experience. People who have studied Ayurvedic and Chinese medicine have been recording and documenting the meridians for over 4,000 years. Over the past 10, I have talked to hundreds of people who have successfully treated themselves and others only by using energy on these meridians.

CHAPTER 17

Leg, Knee, and Hip Injuries

I feel it is important to share about an incident in 1994 that helped open my eyes to old, natural remedies that I had previously dismissed.

I had heard of the healing properties of aloe vera, but tried dozens of aloe products without a noticeable benefit. So I assumed that every aloe product was a scam.

A friend gave me several aloe plants and told me that I would see why it had such a good reputation as a miracle cure. He told me it is mentioned many times in the Bible and touted its healing power. I really respect my friend's knowledge and opinion on health matters, so I politely took the plants home and planted them. I thought that I would try the plants someday, if I ever thought of a reason to use them.

A couple of years went by. I could have benefited from them many times, but never thought about it until it was too late.

One day I got a carpet burn on my knee. I just washed it off without a second thought and went on with my day. In about 3 days, the wound became infected. It never entered my mind to try aloe. I used Neosporin antibiotic ointment and washed and redressed the wound twice a day for several days. My knee got worse. The injury doubled in size and became very painful.

I asked some friends for ideas. Everyone had a different suggestion or remedy. I tried several, but my knee only worsened.

I finally called the friend who had given me the plants. He told me to try them and promised results.

I cut a 1-inch piece, trimmed the stickers from the sides, and butterflied it. I taped it so that it covered about 1/4 of the infected area. The following day I removed it. Not only was the area free of infection, but the healing process was very noticeable. Even the surrounding area seemed somewhat improved.

I then cut a much larger piece and placed it over the entire area. The following day, all of the infection was gone; the healing process was well under way.

I used the plant once more. There was no more tenderness, and it looked like the scar was going away. The redness of the wound was back to its original size.

A year later, the scar was about the size of a silver dollar. It was still noticeable and its coloration was more pink than red. I often wondered whether the scar might have gone away completely if had I used the aloe a few more days. More than a year has passed without any further need for treatment.

Another time, while I visited my friend in Florida, I got a mosquito bite on my leg and scratched it until it started to bleed; it became infected. I used Neosporin, but it kept getting worse. It was several days before I thought of using aloe on it. By the time I did, the wound had grown, was oozing pus, and was very painful. This time I covered the entire infected area with aloe, just before bed. The next morning, the pain and infection had gone. All that was left of the bite was a little red discoloration.

I applied the aloe for 2 more nights and noticed great improvement, but then I quit, thinking it would heal by itself. On the 4th day, the swelling and infection returned. I thought it was because I was only using aloe for 6–7 hours a night, allowing the infection to build up immunity. This happens with any antibiotic. If you do not stay on the drug or a treatment long enough, the infection can return with a stronger resistance. I assumed it was the same with aloe after this experience.

After 9 days, I noticed a little pain and swelling starting to come back. That night, I added a magnet under my leg and slept in my ozone bag. The next morning, the pain and swelling were gone and about 50 percent of the redness had dissipated. The wound continued to respond as I continued this regimen for 2 more days. I was redressing and washing the area 3 times a day, but by the 12th day, my skin was extremely tender from changing the dressing so frequently. I decided to suspend the aloe vera treatment and to leave the wound undressed and exposed to the air.

Most of the tenderness went away after 2 more days. I felt confident that the infection was completely under control, although there was still some discoloration. I treated it for an additional 2 more nights just as a precaution, but after that I only continued to wash the wound morning, noon, and night.

I have a friend in Costa Rica who is a naturopathic doctor. Every morning he blends about a 1-inch-square piece of fresh aloe vera into his juice. He believes that it has regenerated his damaged heart muscle. I do not know if it really did, but I have also started adding aloe to my morning juice.

After my experiences, I believe that the benefits of herbs and other natural nutrients that many manufacturers tout are based on results from live plants. Because I have tried dozens of products with no noticeable benefit, I now feel it is not the plants themselves that have no value, but that processing destroys their beneficial effects.

To accelerate the healing process, I used enzymes, trace minerals, and krill oil to ensure that my body had the nutrition it needed. The magnets provide the energy to reduce pain right away and accelerate healing more rapidly, as that energy speeds up the spin on the electrons. (For a better explanation, please see Chapter 4.)

Some say krill oil is one of the most powerful nutrients ever discovered, and I have found it to be very good. Knowing what I know today, I would have added dimethyl sulfoxide (DMSO), and I would apply it topically as well as take it internally. It breaks up blood clots very rapidly and accelerates healing by reducing inflammation and increasing blood flow.

The human body has some 400 muscles; if these are not used and exercised, they deteriorate. This creates more and more health issues as we age, since little injuries become worse and worse until we can't move well enough to keep lymph fluid moving for overall health.

Even though basic health can be simple, there is a lot to understand about how the parts of the body are interrelated. We are one being, body, mind, and soul; we must address all of these aspects to maintain balance and harmony in our lives to maintain optimum health.

CHAPTER 18

Liver and Minutes to Death

On June 22, 2009, I woke up 2 hours earlier than usual, but since I had answered e-mail until midnight, I didn't want to get up then. I felt uncomfortably full, as if I had eaten too much meat the night before, and a little thirsty. I took 2 tablets of hydrochloric acid (HCl) with a glass of water. I normally only take them at mealtimes to help with my digestion of animal protein (beef, or rarely, pork). The previous day, I had gone jogging first thing in the morning and had felt so good I imagined I would never have another health problem again.

Feeling a bit nauseated, I went back to bed, but a few minutes later, I started throwing up a lot of blood. It continued for a long time; I had never seen this much blood come from anyone who lived. I never had any advance warning, and no pain or even any real discomfort, even while throwing up. It was my first indication that I even had this type of health problem.

As I lay there losing consciousness, feeling certain I would never wake up again, I had time to reflect back on my life and was surprised to find that I was at peace with my Maker and myself.

For the first time, I felt content with my life, and I had absolutely no anxiety about passing on. I thanked God for my blessed life and each wonderful family member I would be leaving, along with many other loved ones.

Just before going to sleep for what I believed would be the last time, I asked God if I still had an unfulfilled purpose or more lessons to learn, I wanted to stay a little longer. I planned to spend the rest of my life doing God's work, and his will, for his glory. I really wanted to leave the world knowing that my life had some meaning and purpose and that I was able to benefit humankind, leaving the world a better place for all. (This has been part of my prayers for the past 20 years.)

A few hours later, I woke up in the hospital and, to my surprise, found myself still breathing. I recall very little of those first few hours, but was told later that the doctor had banded 7 varices, (similar to a varicose vein in my esophagus that ruptured) that were bleeding or about to rupture, and they had given me 8 pints of blood. I have not been able to confirm very much of what took place, as I have never been able to speak to the doctor who performed the operation.

An associate of his came in to see me a couple of days later and asked me if I understood what had happened to me. I said, "I understand that I have cirrhosis, a scarring of the liver; and that when my heart sends blood to my liver to be filtered, it is unable to accept very much of it, creating a blockage which backs up the blood into my esophagus, causing the vessels in my throat to enlarge like varicose veins."

He said it was a very good explanation, and that my condition was stage 4 cirrhosis and untreatable. He said I would be released in a day or two, and he recommend that I use the time to get my affairs in order. He said that at my age I was unlikely to qualify for a liver transplant, which would have been my only option for further treatment.

My first question was, "What can I eat that may help me reverse this?" He said, "There really aren't any dietary guidelines for this condition, other than to stay away from alcohol; other than that, eat about anything you want." I challenged this, because it seemed ridiculous that something in my diet hadn't caused it. He said, "It was most likely caused by an excessive consumption of alcohol when you were younger."

I admitted to drinking in my twenties and thirties, but I had hardly drunk anything for over 20 years. He agreed to have a dietitian from the hospital consult with me before I was released. I had to ask two other doctors and the charge nurse the day of my release before I got a consultation that amounted to someone dropping off a diet for a heart patient and being told it was close enough.

In the hospital, I gained 10 pounds in 4 days, but ate nothing. This is a sign of kidney overload. I had two IV's plugged into me the entire time I was there. Several nurses told me they were a saline solution, a saltwater drip, to keep me hydrated, and nutritional supplements since I could not eat anything for the first 3 days. I thought it was rather ironic to get salt water, since the only other dietary recommendation besides "do not drink alcohol" was "stay on a salt-free diet."

The IV drips blew me up like a balloon to the point where I couldn't even make a fist. I have never heard of anyone gaining 10 pounds in just 4 days without eating anything. On the 3rd day, I was given Jell-O, which is very high in sugar, so I only took a couple of bites. On the day I was released, I was given pork sausage, scrambled eggs, cold hard toast, and a lot of butter and jelly. I did eat the eggs, but that was all. I couldn't believe a hospital would serve a meal of this type for my condition.

Fortunately, I had no appetite; so I wasn't tempted to eat what I know for sure would not be good for me. I was released late that afternoon without eating anything else that day. The first thing I did when I got home was to weigh myself. That's when I realized I had gained 10 pounds.

Nothing sounded good to me to eat, and I had no idea what would be good for me except watermelon. I had been juicing a watermelon a day, for several days before this incident happened and that is the only thing that sounded good to me when I got home from the hospital. Not knowing just what I should eat, I started calling friends for advice. I was soon overwhelmed with suggestions from many doctors, and even some from people I hardly knew.

Ten days after leaving the hospital, I still had not eaten anything except watermelon juice and had lost 25 pounds. I was starting to get very concerned, as I was very glad to lose the 10 pounds of salt water, but the rapid loss of 15 pounds of fat and muscle was scary. I had dropped from 220 pounds to 195 pounds in just 10 days, my cheekbones and eyes were sinking in, and I still had no appetite.

One of my closest friends, Ed from Florida, called that day and said I needed to take my pendulum to the Whole Foods store and start asking it what I should eat. I had piddled around with one on and off for 25 years but never had any faith in it. I thought, why not just flip a coin? Ed walked me through how to use it, and I paid very close attention since I was desperate to stop the rapid weight loss. His information seemed reasonable, but I was still not convinced.

Once I got to Whole Foods I was no longer receiving any information from my pendulum. I tried calling Ed back, but he wasn't available, so I called my friend, Dr. Howard Hagglund, MD, since he routinely uses muscle testing for his own health issues. He is among the most spiritual people I know and really understands how and why this form of testing works. He spent an hour on the phone with me as I walked up and down the aisles testing just about everything in the store.

The only thing it let me eat was goat milk, goat cheese, and quinoa, a very high-protein grain. I had never eaten any of them before, but I was desperate, and watermelon juice was not getting the job done. I just ate quinoa plain, without added seasonings and drank the goat milk for the next couple of days. To my surprise, my weight stabilized the first day at 195 pounds.

I went back to Whole Foods almost every day and spent hours retesting everything, looking for something else I could add to my diet. On the 3rd day, I was able to add sweet potatoes (not yams), but nothing else. I felt confident that I was getting dependable information.

I would hit a wall at times and not get a read at all. One day, my friend Dr. Stephen Daniel (who has a muscle testing DVD course) invited me to come visit him on Maui for a few days. What I learned in a week there made me a believer. I left knowing that I got 100 percent accurate information, and every day since then, I have used what I learned.

What Dr. Daniel taught me has saved me thousands of dollars on products that have no benefit and helps me to find what works before I buy anything. I believe this is a big part of why I continue to feel 20 years old today. Anyone who wishes to better understand this subject can go to www.Quantumtechniques.com; it has information on 17 different testing methods. You don't even need a pendulum. Dr. Daniel's course is very inexpensive, and I feel sure you will do as I have done after seeing the results: tell everyone you know what a fantastic educational tool you have. I have a link to his website if you forget the name of his. www.YourHealthisYourChoice.org

Just 2 months after I became aware of my liver problem, my friend Dr. John Humiston, MD, sent me this e-mail:

Sclerosis is due to long-term inflammation of the liver. Inflammation is a product of either viral infection, fungal infection, or both. If the inflammation is there too long and consistently, it causes the liver cells to slowly die and turn into scar tissue. Once that happens, blood flow is cut off, and the blood backs up either at the base of the esophagus or in the rectum (hemorrhoids) or at the base of the belly button.

Ozone is very good at helping the liver. It is also important to stay on a fungal dietary maintenance program. These measures keep virus and fungus under control. The steady use of alcohol, even though it may be from years ago, can actually be the cause of this. We all need to be aware of this, as a healthy liver is crucial to maintaining our health, and it is probably the most abused; most of us have so little knowledge of its importance and how to take care of it.

Eating a lot of green vegetables and supplementing with essential phospholipids are very good to build cell membrane in the liver. They can be obtained as a supplement along with the other above things mentioned.

None of the liver specialists gave me this type of information, not one of them had any dietary recommendations beyond staying away from alcohol, and my insurance paid them thousands of dollars. This is why I am so disappointed in our health care industry. They don't take the time to educate us about what we can do for ourselves. Dr. Humiston helped me to realize that I needed to start reversing my liver problem, and how important diet was for this.

Dr. Sal D'Onofrio states, "You cannot damage the liver without affecting the other organs, notably your kidneys. Watermelon and its seeds (in watermelon seed tea and seeds in juicing) are one of the main cures for kidney problems."

Watermelons are very high in sugar, which can unbalance pH. I want my pH to be between 7 and 7.2 before juicing a lot of high-sugar fruits and vegetables. Adding a heaping tablespoon of stabilized rice bran to a glass of juice that is high in sugar will dramatically reduce its glycemic effect.

Fortunately, I had three friends who were MD's and several other doctors of other modalities who understood how important diet is for liver issues. They helped guide me to discover what worked to reverse my cirrhosis. Muscle testing with a pendulum was the determining factor in my choice of diet and nutritional supplements.

Energy: I received a spontaneous healing in 1-1/2 hours.

In 7th grade, I learned that we are 99.999 percent *potential* energy. I understood that the distance between an electron and the nucleus in an atom is as great in proportion as the distance between an apple in the United States and an orange in China. The space between electrons is a form of energy consciousness. Energy itself is a form of consciousness. Focused energy creates the particles that make up the universe.

The energy I refer to is not the kind that comes from fossil fuel or other nonrenewable types. It is the unseen and little-known energy that we were never taught about in the United States. It includes magnetic, radionics, orgone, and other types. Some have been used since the beginning of time; they affect our auric field and our cellular structure and have the ability to change us mentally and physically, often in minutes.

Even though I have been aware of several of these types of energies for many years, I have never taken the time to understand how to use any of them. I think I feel, as most people do, that if energy field science were true and important for us to know and understand, it would be on the news. I now realize that it has been in the news many times, and there have been many movies made about it; but like most people, I just write it off as science fiction.

Hearing that a health problem was untreatable inspired me to take a closer look at all options. Christ's saying that "the least among you can do all that I have done and even greater things" had always stood out to me; I believe in the Bible and in Christ, but until my near-death experience, my faith had never really been tested. I never understood the "faith of a mustard seed" or "moving a mountain" parts. However, I am sure I wasn't saved without a purpose, and I am determined to find it. To me, the faith Christ spoke of means that the ability to manifest our health, needs, and desires is within us all. It is up to us to seek out how to use this power for ourselves. I now believe all things are possible, and I had no doubt that I would heal my untreatable liver condition with God's help and guidance.

Our mind has the power to do this using energy. We can also use programmable devices that create this energy. As we learn to capture this energy and put it to use, we will see a world without sickness, diseases, pain, and suffering as we learn to harness the power of our minds.

I visited the Mayo Clinic in Phoenix, Arizona in July 2009. After several tests, I had a consultation with a very attentive doctor. He seemed to have a genuine interest in helping me overcome my cirrhosis, but he offered no hope of any success in reversing it.

In September at a 4 day seminar about the effects of energy on health, I sat in an energy field for an hour and a half and left feeling 100 percent healed. I was not, but it compelled me to devote more time to learning all I can. I will be writing more about this on my websites, www.YourHealthisYourChoice.org and www.DrHealthClub.com.

I had been told to return to the Mayo Clinic every month to have banding done to prevent me from having another life-threatening episode. I did return to Mayo every month for the following year but after the seminar, I did not need the procedure for several months. In the past 2 years it has only needed to be done 2 times and as of January 2012, I was told I do not need to come back for another year as I am doing so well.

In February 2010, my doctor was excited to see the improvement in my blood work. He said, "Excuse me, I need a second opinion for this," and left the room. He returned in a few minutes with the doctor in charge of my liver evaluation for a transplant. Both asked what I had been doing, because my blood tests indicated my liver was functioning normally even though the cirrhosis is still showing up on the CAT scan. They said, "We have never seen that before."

The doctor said, "Today we are here to learn, and we want to know what you have been doing to accomplish this." For the next hour, I did my best to explain that it was a combination of products and energy. I went into my story that we are 99.999 percent energy and how much distance there is between electrons and nuclei in an atom. Energy holds all particles together as electrons revolve around the nucleus just as earth revolves around the sun; our solar system is in similar motion.

Just as magnetic energy's effect on our body's energy fields plays a big part in our health, so does the power of prayer, which is energy as well. The radionic energy, scalar energy, and zero-point energy in the wands that Dr. Hagglund brought to my attention recently, are other forms that play an important part in our lives and our health. Most schools don't teach us about them, so for the most part, we have little understanding of their influence.

Electromagnetic radiation is another form of energy that few were aware of until Senator Ted Kennedy died from brain cancer.

He felt that the cancer was caused by cell phone energy, according to several news programs I listen to, and I agree. There are probably other harmful sources of energy as well. High-tension power lines, cell phone towers, the electromagnetic energy emitted by the power lines in our homes are all forms of subtotal (you don't see, feel or hear it) energy that could affect our lives and our health.

Many realize that a microwave creates heat, because it reverses the spin on the electrons and destroys the nutritional value of much of our food. Few realize that microwaves were outlawed in Russia for many years now. The Russian government paid for research and analysis on them, realized the harm they do, and outlawed them.

When I learned about the negative effects of cell phone energy, I did my best to protect myself from it. I have used EMR blockers on my cell phones for more than 10 years. I have not used a microwave at all for 5 years. To date, I have not noticed negative effects of EMR on my brain. I have seen the thermal photography used to check this firsthand, so I know EMR blockers work.

Here is a list of what I have been using and doing to heal my "untreatable" liver cirrhosis:

1. Diet. It is critical for good health, but there is no need to be fanatic about it. No matter what your health issues are, until you get them under control, diet and internal cleansing should be your first consideration, at least for a few months.

2. The single most important thing was the pendulum I use to test everything I put in my mouth and to protect myself from EMR.

3. ASEA: I cannot say for sure how much it benefited my liver, but I took it for about a year (which included my visit

to the Mayo Clinic when their doctors were so impressed with my condition).

4. Optimum D-Tox: This is a natural whole food product that has many nutrients that aid the body in healing itself.

5. Enzymes: Vitalzym has the largest combination of enzymes in their formula that I am aware of, along with added ingredients to allow them to work synergistically. Dr. D'Onofrio says Neprinol is stronger, and I plan to start trying it.

6. Amino acids: Sometimes I have had noticeable results in just 15 minutes.

When the liver is not functioning right and doesn't filter out the ammonia from protein fermentation in the large intestine, it goes to your brain and causes ammonia intoxication, with symptoms similar to Alzheimer's. It can last several hours, during which you cannot have a coherent conversation. Within 15 minutes of taking my amino acids, transamination would occur: the nitrogen in the ammonia would bond with the amino acids, turning into glucose. I would regain clarity of thought, and often, a noticeable improvement in my eyesight in a very short time. The amino acid I used was one of the very things my pendulum allowed me to take.

I have since found that bee pollen and sea kelp are a very good source of all 22 amino acids, and it is from a natural, whole food. Pollen from a local beekeeper can provide an added benefit to your immune system and prevent or reduce allergies to local plants. It is quite inexpensive for the benefit you get. Bee pollen has many other nutrients and potential health benefits as well.

In addition, prayer motivates me to share my story and to give others hope in reversing their health problems as I have done. I do not consider myself to be exceptionally smart, just very determined and open to receive God's guidance. The picture "Footprints in the Sand" had a real impact on me the first time I saw it; it hangs right by my bed now. It is the last thing I see when I go to bed and say my prayers and is the first thing I see when I wake up. I tear up when I reflect on the saying, "My precious, precious child, I love you and would never leave you. During your times of trial and suffering, when you see only one set of footprints, it was then that I carried you."

I received the blessing of forgiveness in 1974 and realized that I would be forgiven as I forgive others, and I would be judged as I judge others. This changed my life. I pray every day for the ability to continue to do God's work and his will, for his glory. I live my life in gratitude, thanking God for the opportunities to serve him and be a benefit to humanity as I share my stories of success about my many health challenges.

In May 2011, I went to Idaho to work on my book where I would have few interruptions and distractions. I didn't take a lot of supplements or other things I have at home, and I often found myself eating out and buying things I knew I shouldn't eat for snacks while I was writing. I still felt great, but my diet continued to regress, and I found myself often eating like I did when I was in my twenties. At home 4 weeks later, I continued to eat badly and I woke up June 1 feeling uncomfortably full. This time there was no bleeding or any other negative effect, but I believed it was related to my liver damage.

I had been putting off working on the liver chapter, as I needed to go over hundreds of pages of my notes and doctors' tests and reports. Up to now, I had not wanted to deal with all that. Now I had a reason to dig back through it all, looking for answers to repair the recent damage I had done to my liver and other organs with my dietary abuse.

Even though my liver had been functioning normally, according to my Mayo Clinic blood work, I think now it would still show as normal. I still have much of the scarring, so my liver isn't like new even though I felt like it was.

To get back on track, I modified my diet again:

1. I drank a quart of organic apple juice per day.

2. I had juiced watermelon with stabilized rice bran for breakfast for a few weeks.

3. For the first week I also drank pure water, treated to add energy.

4. I ate nothing but fresh fruits and vegetables for a few days, undercooked in waterless cookware. I added little or no seasoning, but added a little flax seed, rice bran, coconut oil, or extra virgin olive oil after cooking.

5. Other than the above oils, I consumed no other fat for the first few weeks. Then I added a little organic butter and just a very little sea salt. (I use only Real Salt from the caverns close to Salt Lake City, Utah. I believe this is the purest salt available; it comes from underground, is free of contamination, and has not been exposed to the environment for thousands of years.)

6. I followed Dr. D'Onofrio's protocol for a liver cleanse (see Chapter 20).

7. I followed his protocol for a coffee enema's after the 6th day.

On the 7th day, I felt like I never had my liver bother me in the first place.

I was very surprised to see just how resilient my body really was. I have had many great experiences over the past 20 years, but I was amazed at how quickly cleanses turned this problem around. However, I remained on this diet for several more weeks.

Most importantly, I learned that I must still have cirrhosis. Otherwise I could have continued to abuse my liver far more than before.

My latest trip to the Mayo Clinic was in January 2012, and my liver was fine. I had my prostate checked, along with my kidneys and bladder, and there was nothing noticeable to report on any tests.

I really do love feeling 20 years old once again, and I am looking forward to the next 100 years, still feeling 20. I believe that is possible with today's technology. Just think how much more we will learn in the next 10 years alone! Our knowledge is growing exponentially with our access to computers.

Live in love and light.

CHAPTER 19

Nose Cancer / Skin Cancer

By 2000, although I had occasional relapses, my general health had continued to improve since 1991, but I had been watching a red spot on the tip of my nose for a few years. It would fade for months and then reappear out of the blue. It wasn't blotchy, discolored, or mottled like a picture of melanoma in a medical book, but I was suspicious of it just the same.

Over the next few years when the spot was visible, I would ask doctors at the health trade shows if it looked cancerous and whether I should worry about it. Several dozen doctors over several years all said no, it did not appear to be melanoma.

I would also ask alternative healers, people who understood how energy affects physical and emotional health. I was becoming more interested in energy technology using quantum techniques (QT), an advanced form of energy medicine. The intent of QT is to heal chronic illness and/or to remove emotional blockages using vibrational frequencies.

Think of your body as a computer, where each of its 10 major organs has a hard drive. Emotional, physical, or even food trauma can disconnect any of these organs from the "terminal" the body. QT brings that connection back using a series of "healing codes" so the body can repair itself from any type of trauma. Based on some tests, the QT practitioners were sure that the red spot on my nose was indeed cancerous.

Another 6 months had gone by, and I was annoyed because the spot on my nose had not faded as usual. I was not alarmed, but thought it was time to call a doctor to solve the mystery. I had a dermatologist examine the spot. He didn't believe it was cancer, but he ordered a biopsy just to make sure. A week later, I got a call to come in his office to discuss the results. To his surprise, they had come back positive for melanoma. We discussed options, but he recommended surgical removal. He said it would probably take close to a quarter inch off the tip of my nose. "What is the lesser of two evils?," I thought. Reluctantly, I agreed.

The procedure left a very noticeable scar. I was told that if it bothered me, it would be no problem to have it repaired. I didn't give that much thought. When it was totally healed, it was not that bad, and, except for taking notes on it, I pretty much forgot about it.

Three years later, the spot returned and then faded. A year later, it was permanent once again. I was frustrated that the operation had not been successful. I tried tablets and salves from health stores, but nothing was effective beyond 2 or 3 months. The spot returned, and I never figured out why.

This was before I met Jim Humble, Dr. William Hitt, and Dr. John Humiston in Mexico. I had a small house on the beach there, and on one of my trips I visited a friend who shares my interest in alternative medicine. He told me about the "Hoxsey Clinic" just across the border in Tijuana. It uses a combination of diet, vitamins, minerals, and herbs to treat people and animals with a black Indian salve. The clinic has a long and controversial past in treating cancer, but I was open to anything at this point!

Early in 2007, I met with Dr. Gutierrez at the clinic (its real name is the Bio-Medical Center). I was very impressed with the modern facilities and the staff. Everyone speaks English, and they make waiting very comfortable. The only times I have been to a doctor's office where I looked forward to sitting out front and waiting have been at the Hitt Center and at the Hoxsey Clinic, both in Mexico. I have met some of the most interesting people from all over the world while waiting to see the doctor and many with incredible stories of their success from the treatment they have received.

They have several videos about Dr. Hoxsey and what the FDA did to him, and how his knowledge has survived despite incredible hardship. I was fascinated with his story and the success of the Hoxsey treatment. After my treatment, I went back to the waiting room and spent 2 more hours talking to people and reading more about this remarkable man and this incredible place. The time and expense of my visit was worth it just for the history lessons.

The program at the clinic has saved thousands, and I have been blessed to speak with dozens of them over the past few years. I stop by from time to time just to sit in the waiting room to listen and learn. I have never found another clinic or group of doctors who work from the heart and have so much to offer patients except Drs. Hitt and Humiston (who also worked in Tijuana). Unfortunately, Dr. Hitt died in August, 2010 at the age of 84 in the United States after being treated in Mexico. His death was attributed to an infection that caused gastrointestinal bleeding due to complications from a hip replacement operation done in the United States. I was fortunate enough to have visited with him at his clinic a few weeks before his passing. He had been full of life and was still working right up to his death. He was looking forward to the operation so he could be of more service to his patients. When Dr. Humiston called to tell me of Dr. Hitt's passing, I felt I had lost a real friend; and I know the world lost an incredible man.

Many doctors have treated cancer successfully for nearly 100 years or more, but many have been jailed or their lives have been destroyed. Royal Raymond Rife, Dr. Hoxsey, and dozens of others have suffered from the FDA's abuse of power. I do not mean to make this so political, but I just can't seem to help myself sometimes. I have seen the fear in so many people's eyes while they tell their stories of dealing with the FDA.

The staff took several tests along with some X-rays; and soon Dr. Gutierrez and I were looking at them on a monitor. He explained that I had cancer on the tip of my nose and that the root had grown in on each side of the cartilage. He recommended using black salve.

I told him that I had already tried several types but saw no results. He said there are many knockoffs on the market, but he has never seen any of them work like the Hoxsey salve. I was still reluctant to accept this, since the treatment cost $4,000, but it came with a lifetime guarantee. You could come back as often as necessary.

About that time Liz Jonas stopped by to see how I was doing. She is the sister of Mildred Nelson, a registered nurse who had worked for Dr. Hoxsey in the 1950s. Liz was old enough to be retired, but chose to keep working at the clinic. She seemed younger than I, although we are about the same age. She is still filled with the excitement of being of service to others. She immediately impressed me, and she took the time to listen to my concerns.

I was very concerned about ending up with a large scar on the end of my nose.I told her about my experiences, my many health challenges, and that I had been documenting everything for15 years at that time. She was very patient and listened intently. I explained that I wanted to write a book about my experiences and successes. I felt it would benefit many people, but I thought it would be more effective without a very noticeable, large part of my nose missing.

She just laughed and said, "Look at the end of my nose. Do you see a scar?" I could just barely see a tiny scar on its tip, just about where my spot was. She said, "This is why I am here. I had the same problem many years ago. I went to doctors all over the United States, and all they wanted to do was cut my nose off."

She said, "That never made sense to me. I know it wasn't my nose's fault it had cancer! I realized it was just a symptom of an underlying problem that needed to be addressed, and I had no medical education at that time. I came here to see my sister, took her treatment, and realized that she really understood not only how to cure cancer but many, if not most, other diseases as well."

"I was so impressed with what I learned and the results of her treatment that I never left. My sister needed my help because of my business background, and saw how I could help not only her, but many others as well. As you can see, I am still here."

This was not a sales pitch; no one could be that good an actress. I was so moved by her story that I opted to have the procedure done right then. I really liked it there. Liz's attitude was so contagious that the whole staff had a similar positive and helpful attitude; it seemed everyone was dedicated to being of service to others. Later when I would visit and Liz was there, she always made time to chat and teach me more about what they do, how they do it, and why she can't bring herself to retire. Once, she said, "When God blesses one with the knowledge to be of service to humanity and him at the same time, how could anyone quit?"

I called Liz recently to see how she is doing. She was still working and running the clinic as of October 2011. She still sounds full of life and filled with the excitement of being of service to others. I have so much respect and admiration for her and what she has accomplished in helping others overcome their health problems. She is such an inspiration that I want to do the same. I hope my book will help many to understand that only the body can heal itself and that health can be simple.

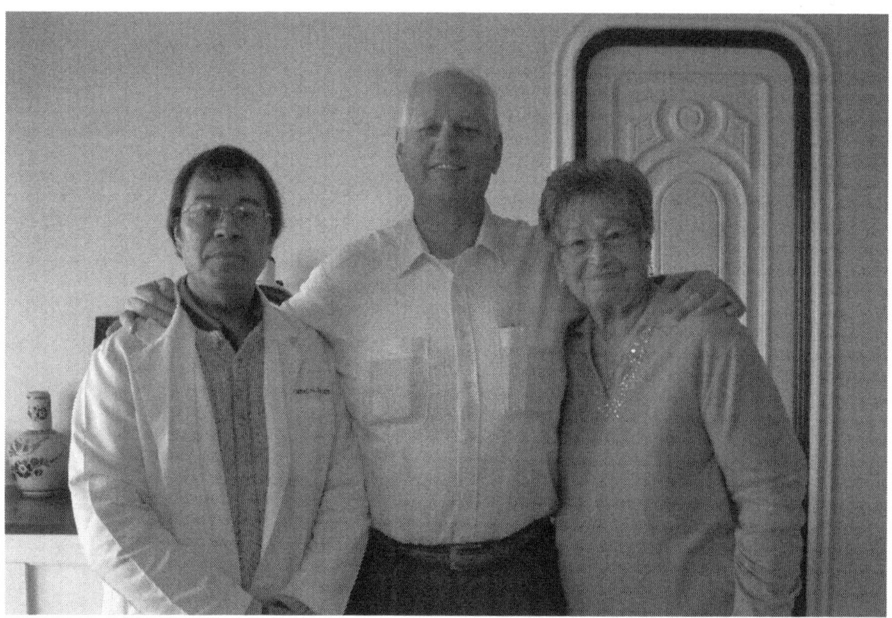

This picture was taken at the Hoxsey Clinic just minutes before Dr. Gutierrez started his procedure. (L to R: Dr. Gutierrez, Dennis Richard, Liz Jones)

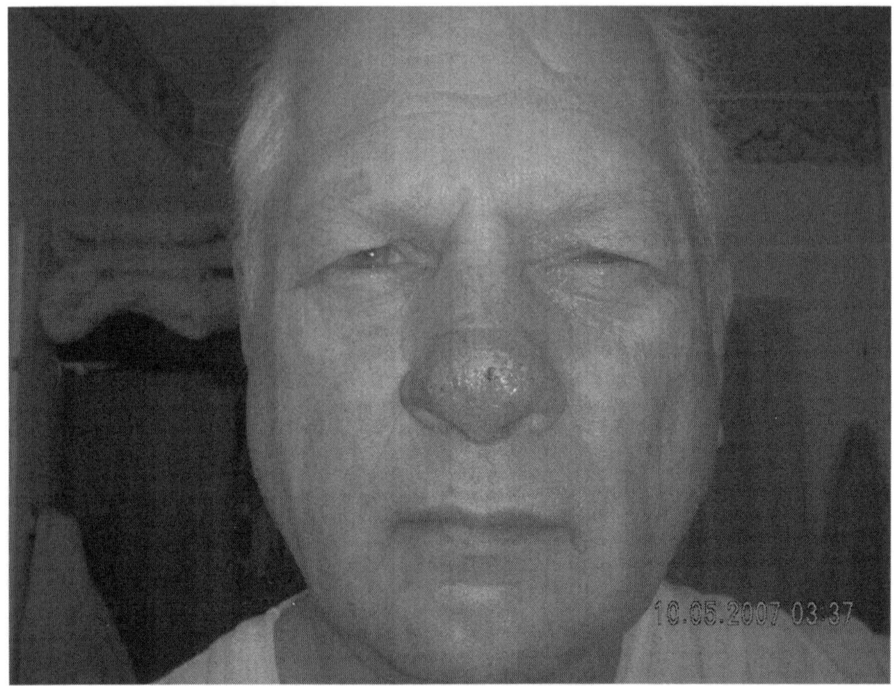

BEFORE: Just after this, Dr. Gutierrez dabbed the Hoxsey black salve on my nose.

When Dr. Gutierrez applied the salve, the pain was almost unbearable. I have a very low tolerance to pain. At the time, I thought the salve seemed to burn the cancer out, along with some of the surrounding healthy tissue. 5 years later, I think it only affected the cancerous tissue. The pain lasted about 15 minutes but slowly became less intense and the burning sensation subsided, but it was quite uncomfortable for a while longer. When the pain diminished, I saw two large, burn-like areas, one on each side of the tip of my nose. I had a couple of months of healing ahead of me.

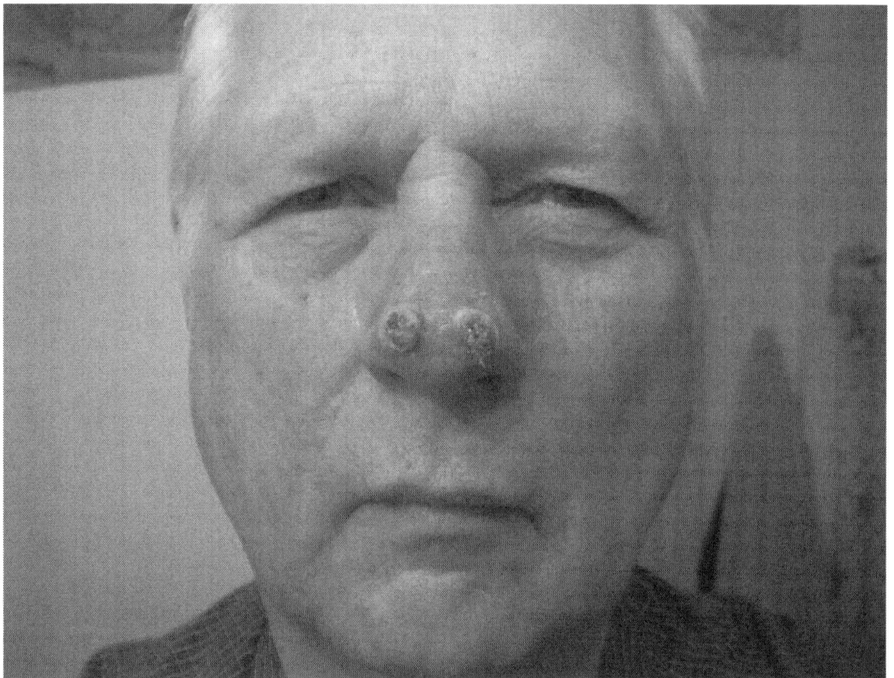

AFTER: At home, a few days later

The craters scabbed over and seemed very large. It took a couple of months to heal completely while I washed and redressed my nose and put a yellow salve on the two burn areas twice a day. After just a few days, one of the scabs came off in the shower while I was washing my nose. The pain felt like it had when the doctor put the salve on the first time. It burned, but it also it felt like someone had punched me in my nose at the same time. The pain was so intense I could not finish my shower. I went to the mirror to see how bad it was. The crater was very deep. I thought it would always look hideous, and I realized that tears were running down my cheek. These were not tears of emotion but tears of intense pain. The pain ran from the tip of my nose right into my brain.

It took about 15 minutes to clean my nose up. I stopped the bleeding in a couple of minutes with a small neodymium magnet.

The pain subsided, and I dressed the injury and re-taped the magnet on the outside of the dressing before I was able to finish the rest of my shower. Once again, I was amazed at how fast the magnets worked to stop the pain and bleeding. I left the small magnet on for several days, and it accelerated the healing.

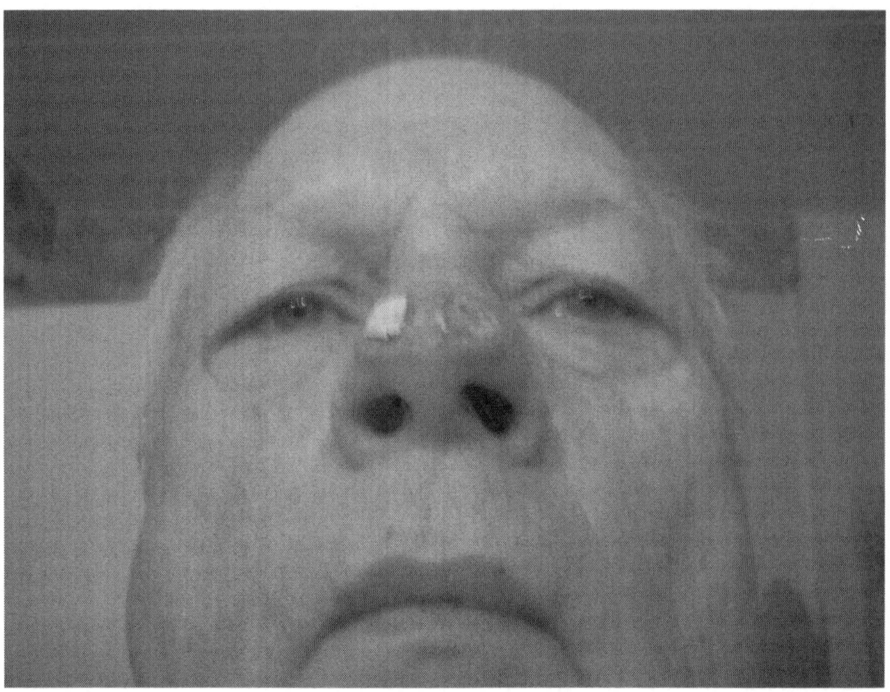

Another scab replaced the old one in a few days, but the one that came off first left a larger pockmark for a few months. It became the smaller of the two scars within a year, and I think the magnet made the difference. When both scabs finally came off, I had two very large craters in the end of my nose. It was scary-looking at first, but soon I felt they became much less noticeable. Four years later I still have noticeable scars, but when I tell my story, most people comment that they barely noticed them.

Early in 2009, the red spot came back. I called the same doctor who had performed my first operation in the States. Another biopsy was done; and once again, my results returned positive for melanoma. I could not bring myself to have more of my nose removed without trying some other new cancer remedies that I had run across.

If I couldn't find anything else that worked, I would definitely opt to go back to the Hoxsey Clinic before having my nose cut again. I felt so confident that the Hoxsey protocol worked completely to burning the cancer out of my nose, but I was not diligent in following their diet and taking the liquid product they gave me at the time. Before I had their procedure on my nose, I could feel the cancer attached to the cartilage in my nose when I touched it. After the scabs were gone and I could feel my nose, I no longer felt that deep-seated attachment; I was sure it was all gone at the time. If I don't find another way to deal with this successfully, I will go back and follow their instructions to the letter the next time.

I had been using Sodium Chlorite (MMS) for other health issues along with several other things, and was very surprised to find the cancer had come back. It is obvious there is no silver bullet; however, I have received a great deal of benefit from Sodium Chlorite (MMS), Molecula Silver, and other things I have tried. Yet none of them prevented the cancer from coming back. I still believe that Sodium Chlorite (MMS) has the potential to reverse most types of cancer, since I have spoken to hundreds of people who said it worked for them; it just does not work 100 percent of the time for all forms of cancer.

Before I was willing to consider submitting to another operation or going back to the Hoxsey Clinic, I wanted to find something less intrusive. When cleansing my colon with Optimum D-Tox in 2009, I got a very surprising benefit. I went from a 42" to a 36" waist in a 6-month period while only losing 10 pounds of body fat. So I started using another product from the same company in the summer of 2010. I added their Esseniac Herbal Tea in with the Optimum D-Tox. These two products are said to work synergistically with the body's immune system.

I am happy to report that the red spot went away within a couple of months, and there has been no reoccurrence to date. In January 2011, I went back to the Mayo Clinic in Phoenix for my liver cirrhosis checkup (read about this remarkable visit in my

January 15, 2012 newsletter at my website, www.YourHealthis YourChoice.ORG)!

Finally, I would like to include a contribution from Dr. Sal D'Onofrio from September 2011:

The object of Gerson's highly successful program is to enable parenteral digestion of tumors, elimination through the liver via the bile ducts, and a return to normal homeostasis. This program was successfully used in over 50 terminal, inoperable, "given up to die" cases. The program worked, because it addressed the causes which are lack of oxygen to the tissues and removal of toxic wastes causing free radical damage, thus weakened cells and boosting the immune system.

Oxygen is carried by alkaline blood. Blood is alkalinized by minerals from vegetable juices, soups, some fruits, and the rest of my strict diet.(The oxygen in Sodium Chlorite (MMS) aids in cancer programs.)

The liver is cleansed and detoxed along with the blood dialysis result of coffee enemas. (The Optimum D-Tox cleanses the liver as well).

The immune system is maximized by the rich, biologically available nutrients from the diet. It is also now able to target pathogens, because the diet is 100 percent digestible.

Instead a Cell Mediated Response can now happen and target the fungus, bacteria, and virus that are part of the cancer process. The cancer process can only occur in acid blood (mineral deficient) that cannot carry enough oxygen which prevents cells from straying from their natural order of mitosis to uncontrolled cellular division known as cancer.

CHAPTER 20

Energy, Colonics, Parasites, and Dysentery

My first experience with a colonic was in the 1970s with Dr. Ritter, DC. He was addressing the lower back problems that had plagued me through most of my career on the fire department and the chronic kidney and bladder infections I often had from the 1960s through the 1980s. He assured me that a series of colonics would cleanse my colon and remove the stress from my immune system, allowing it to better deal with chronic kidney infections.

After a series of them, I was surprised to find that they did work as the doctor said. I did not have any kidney infections for many years; however, you know the saying "out of sight, out of mind." Well, I never realized the benefit of those colonics until many years later when I started experiencing other health problems. By1991 when I retired, I was so sick; several friends and individuals brought colonics back to my attention. I started on another series of these cleanses (as discussed in chapter 11).

At the time of my retirement, I could hardly carry on a conversation without forgetting the point. I was unable to think logically, much less follow a protocol to help myself. After a series of IV chelation therapies, my mind came back and I was able to start thinking normally again. After some analysis, I realized that they were a form of cleansing the circulatory system and the brain. It made sense to go back to colon cleansing and colonics again.

On a trip to the Dominican Republic and Haiti in the summer of 2010, I seemed to have contracted dysentery. 6 weeks after it had started and stopped several times, I realized it was getting very serious. I have had many bouts with dysentery, but nothing like this. When I had stomach problems or loose bowels in the 1940s, my mother would give me Paregoric; within a few minutes (or at most a few hours), I would be fine. Paregoric had a form of narcotic in it and the FDA took it off the market back in the 1950s.

On June 11, 2010, I had dinner at a nice restaurant at a hotel in Barahona, Dominican Republic, a few miles from Jim Humble's Mission; I had a very good chicken dish with a salad. I have probably spent several cumulative years traveling in Mexico and other countries far more "third world;" and I know better than to eat salads. I was with others who had been eating them there for several days with no ill effects, and it really sounded good, so I had one as well.

The next morning, I woke up and ran to the bathroom, and again an hour later. Then I went to my class at Jim Humble's Mission retreat. I mixed up a 6-drop dose of Sodium Chlorite (MMS) and took it on an empty stomach. It seemed a little hard on my stomach, but I felt it got the job done. By 8:00 a.m., when they served breakfast, I thought my problem was gone and I was very hungry.

I had gone on the trip without my pendulum "pendant" that I use to test what I eat. If not for that, I doubt I would have this story to tell. Everything always happens for the best; our most memorable learning experiences are often the most painful.

By that afternoon, I was feeling much better but was getting hungry; Jim suggested boiled white rice. I had no further problems Saturday night or all day Sunday. I had a little chicken and some vegetables for dinner. Many times over the next few weeks, I was sure I was over the problem, but it continued to plague me for months.

In July, I ate eggs for breakfast for the first time in over 3 weeks, and it all started over again. I could not believe it. Fortunately, my good friend Doug Widdifield would be the guest health care professional on the educational conference call I would be hosting the next morning. He spoke about his 30 years of work with the yucca plant. He used it and developed it as an agricultural product for 10 years when he recognized that it might be a beneficial supplement for others. When he gave it to his father, he quickly saw improvement in a health problem. Then he gave it to friends and family, following the guidelines of a doctor who had also been researching yucca.

His remarkable product caught the attention of the Chinese government. They would spend $4,000,000 to research Optimum D-Tox, and it became the first herbal product in Chinese history allowed to be imported. To date there have been only two, and Doug is the developer and manufacturer of both.

Doug explained how Optimum D-Tox benefits the digestive system. I had 5 emergency bowel movements while hosting the call from the throne in just 2 hours. After the call, I found the bottle of Optimum D-Tox sitting in my cupboard. I had not been taking it for some time.

Using my pendulum to see if I should take it, it showed a very strong yes. It also indicated I should take 14 drops. I was hesitant to take that much, since Doug had said I should take only 8, 3 times a day, at the most. I took the 14 drops, 3 times a day after a confirming opinion from a second pendulum I sometimes use. I had no ill effects from taking the extra amount, and I have been pleased with the results. I only took the extra amount for a short time; my pendulum had me drop back to the recommended amount.

When I tested about taking Sodium Chlorite (MMS) with the Optimum D-Tox, the pendulum said to maintain a 2-hour separation between them. I am happy to report that I was just fine the rest of the day. I continued to take the Optimum D-Tox, alternated with the Sodium Chlorite (MMS) every 2 hours for a few months.

On July 24, I was not able to get away from the toilet until noon. I took 14 more drops of the Optimum D-Tox at 5:00 a.m. and 6 drops of Sodium Chlorite (MMS) at 7:00 a.m., and I was still hitting the toilet every hour or two. I checked with my pendulum every time. I repeated the same again 4 hours later, and then I followed that with a 6-drop Sodium Chlorite (MMS) enema. By noon, I had it under control and was very hungry. I normally have very little appetite while the bugs are active.

Dr. Hitt and Dr. Humiston told me that fungus can manipulate the brain's chemistry to make you crave what it wants to eat. It seems that whatever these superbugs are, they have the same ability; I have repeated the cycle several times in 6 weeks. The pendulum told me that there is more than one type of superbug, but I don't have the education to figure out which they are. The pendulum only responds to yes or no questions; there are likely hundreds of different types of pathogens, and I couldn't ask about each by name.

Some of the other things I took were plain goat kefir and yogurt, probiotics, iodine, Esseniac Herbal Tea (a product based on the formula to make essiac tea), vitamins K and D, and several types of herbal blends for the colon. I often checked to see if I could take amino acids, as I felt sure I needed them to help reverse lost muscle mass, but the answer was most often no. I assume that some of these superbugs thrive on protein or at least something in that particular product. Before I had this problem, it was rare that the pendulum gave me a "no" for any of them.

That evening when I got home from a health show, I asked my pendulum if I could eat some more quinoa and goat yogurt; and it said yes. Once again, I was back on the pot in about 15 minutes, and it was all water; I just couldn't believe it. I asked if I should take more Sodium Chlorite (MMS), and it said no, so I asked if I should take the D-Tox, and it said yes, so I took 14 drops. My stomach settled down, and I felt much better.

At 6:00 p.m. I was getting hungry, so I asked the pendulum if I could eat some squash, and it said yes; then I asked if it would cause me to have another bowel movement, and it said yes. I then asked if this would help me get rid of some of the bad bugs causing the problem. This helped to clarify my understanding of how to ask questions, so my problem had provided an opportunity to learn. I hope this lengthy explanation helps you as well. I see it as another blessing in life's learning experiences.

Later in July when I felt very bad, I went to my friend Linda Hathaway, who put me on her Eternale and Indigo machine, doing biofeedback on me for 3 hours. I felt ready to go back to work when I left. I am so thankful I kept my appointment that morning, because I started the day feeling about 50 percent of my normal self, and it increased to about 90 percent by the end of it.

The Indigo Biofeedback system finds and detects over 11,000 stress areas in the biological energy fields of the human body. It constantly measures and balances those stressors at incredible speed. Each of us has different stressors. The machine only measures what is needed and what someone's field wants, then reduces stress for that time. Biofeedback retraining energy fields of the visible body to remember their baseline or balance. The Eternale is an automated system that uses the same technology as the INDIGO.

Electromagnetic stressors, or "perverse energies," are just one type of stress that shows on the visible body but which we cannot see with the naked eye. The Eternale works on hair, skin, and nails, and builds self-esteem. It uses Solfeggio tones (6 sound energy frequencies) with background music to ease stress in the mind with guided self-imagery to create a strong foundation for making healthy choices in eating habits, exercise, and reaction to outside stress. The Eternale can harmonize the body's energy fields and help to create a feeling of youthfulness. I used it almost every day for 17 days. It helped me to sleep comfortably, and I woke each morning feeling great. I know most healing takes place in a state of relaxed sleep.

While working with the energy, I was taking colonics as well; I have had over 50 colonics in 40 years. By now, I know how it feels when toxins are expelling. The water temperature feels relatively comfortable up to quite hot. With this new series, I felt a

4–5-degree rise in temperature. On the second, with the Sodium Chlorite (MMS), the temperature felt 5–10 degrees hotter almost continually. At times, it was comparable to the feeling of eating a whole jalapeño that had not lost any fire on its way out. But even after several colonics, the diarrhea did not stop for more than a few days.

I host one conference call a week now, every Tuesday night from 5:45 to 8:00 p.m. PST.(If you would like to call in, the number is 712-432-3100 and the code is 388191.) I had Georgia Cold scheduled more than a month in advance, and at the time, I had no idea how badly I would need her information. It came at a critical time; my dysentery was worsening steadily. I was always confident that I could overcome any health challenge with what I had learned, but I did not take dysentery seriously enough. I knew that millions have died from it—many thousands during World War II. Although I have never known anyone who had, and I never had it last more than 2 or 3 days, this episode got me down.

Fortunately, I now had many resources, hundreds of doctors and health care professionals, of whom I can ask advice. I called a few and integrated their suggestions into what I had been doing. Nevertheless, I was still losing the battle; it had lasted 7 weeks, no matter what I tried. I even increased fiber in my diet with psyllium, wheat, oat and rice bran, and rice fiber, adding it to what little I had been eating. This helped a little, but it still was not getting the job done.

Georgia Cold is a registered nurse from Montana. She has an extensive background in allopathic medicine, but she ended up becoming a colon hydrotherapist, because she found that it worked far better than anything else she had learned about health. I spoke to her at length for the first time ever just an hour before the conference call, and was impressed. I have often mentioned that I believe I lead a guided life, as I am one of the few people I know out of the thousands I talk to who have no plan. Many others tend to try to create a plan to make life work out the way they want it to. I am happy living life day to day, enjoying every minute and accepting what is and whatever happens. I am cool with being in the moment. I hear many people talk about being in the moment and enjoying it, but few can truly do it. It seems just a natural way of life for me. I want to experience all of life's lessons, and I am eager to learn from them all. Learning from T. Harv Eker that "nothing has meaning but the meaning you give it" really made an impact on my life.

Before the call with Georgia Cold, I felt colonics would help and had taken several in the past few weeks with only temporary benefit. After speaking to her for an hour before our scheduled conference call, I felt sure she had all the answers I needed to eradicate the super bugs causing this problem.

During the call, Ms. Cold and I discussed why nothing I had been doing for the past 2 months had worked for me permanently. Because my lack of diligence in continuing Sodium Chlorite (MMS) had allowed the bugs to gain strength, they had buried their offspring in the layers of plaque in my intestines where there is no blood supply. They could survive and continue to play havoc in my digestive system. The protocol of my local colon hydrotherapist had not gotten rid of plaque allowing for a protected breeding ground, and the bugs had become acclimated. That's why it had had no long-term benefit.

Georgia pointed out there are two primary types of colon hydrotherapy units. The type that most use (including my local hydro therapist) are referred to as "open," meaning that there is a 2-lb. positive pressure; you simply eliminate the water as you feel the urge. The second type has a positive 2 lbs. of pressure as it fills your intestines and a 1-lb. negative pressure as you eliminate or evacuate your colon. Georgia has both types, but she says she gets much better results with the latter.

In addition, she starts her clients on a pre-diet cleanse to condition the colon to maximize results. She gets much better results than the usual colon hydrotherapist does with her Healing Waters cleanse. It is a guided juice fasting program that incorporates a combination of carrots, beets, celery, and apples with the traditional Master Cleanse. Each ingredient does something different within the body. The celery breaks down plaque within the body and aids sleep. The beets clean the blood, liver, and colon. The carrots act as antioxidants to keep toxins and free radicals at bay, and the apples contain malic acid that gets into the core of the plaque buildup and mixes with the lemon in the Master Cleanse to loosen and soften the plaque itself.

The cayenne pepper in the Master Cleanse acts as a stimulant to keep the intestines awake and moving throughout the fasting process. Maple syrup or molasses keeps the blood sugar stable, so that even diabetics can benefit from this cleanse. A colonic is given every day of the 5 days of juicing. As the plaque begins to loosen, it is imperative to remove it with colon therapy. You will watch sheets of it, sometimes as long as 4–6 feet, expel from your body over the 5 days.

The procedure is done in a safe, comfortable environment with a trained colon therapist. Warm filtered water is introduced into the colon at a very slow rate. There should be no pain as the procedure removes what has been stuck in the intestines over a lifetime. It lasts between 45 and 60 minutes. The therapist monitors both the temperature and the pressure of the filtered water, as it irrigates the bowel. If you suffer from constipation, diarrhea, backache, loss of concentration, indigestion, headaches, yeast infections, allergies, insomnia, gas, bloating, frequent colds or infections, general aches and pains, low energy, skin rashes, or a whole host of other conditions, you need to experience this cleanse.

About 70 others from many different states (as well as several from Canada) discussed all this on our call. Georgia did a great job of explaining many of the benefits of being diligent about cleansing the colon. After the call was over, I scheduled Georgia's series of colonics for the following week. To contact her, go to www.healingwatersforhealth.com. This experience was worth the 2,400-mile drive to me.

I went back to the Dominican Republic to attend some more of Jim Humble's classes. On this second trip I went for 3 weeks with no problem at all. It returned once I got home, but it was minor in comparison. I used mostly just Sodium Chlorite (MMS), taking it both orally and rectally, along with slippery elm and a few other herbs. It brought it under control in a day or two, and I thought that Sodium Chlorite (MMS) was getting the job done for good this time, because I had finally cleaned my colon adequately to remove the bugs' breeding ground. It seemed I should have taken more of the colonics while I was in Montana, since I know that when I left, there was still a lot more in me.

In December 2010, my problem started again, and I soon realized it could become life threatening again. I tried to figure out what to do. I tried not eating for the rest of the day, but the problem was still there in the morning. I repeated my protocol and went back to bed thinking that I had I brought the problem back to haunt me with a bad diet. I realized that several things might have contributed to this re-infestation:

1. At Thanksgiving, I ate many things I knew I should not, such as sweets, breads, and other carbs. They turn to sugar and feed many pathogens.

2. Increased eating of cheese and other dairy products.

3. Adding eggs back into my diet several times a week. Eggs foster rapid growth of many species of bacteria.

I have recovered for a few days to a month or so several times now; each time I think it is gone for good, but then I start eating eggs, and it comes back again. I was in one of these cycles when I bought the Photon Genie in December 2010 for my prostate, but it didn't enter my mind to try it for dysentery problem.

However, since I slept with the Genie's probes, the problem has gone away. I suspected that the Genie may have helped, so I started eating eggs every day again to see if it would come back. At this point, I do not feel comfortable saying for sure, but it could be possible. I thought $3000 was a lot to pay for the Genie, but I spent a lot more on other things trying to get over the dysentery. I felt it was life threatening on a few occasions and I had no confidence that allopathic medicine could help, so the money was not that important under the circumstances. I believe this equipment should be available in every hospital and doctor's office in America.

By January 2012, I was very happy to report that I did not have further problems with dysentery over the previous 11 months and ate eggs nearly every day.

Benefits I have derived from energy, sleeping better, clarity of thought, and the reduction of all stress:

Restoring missing cellular communication helps the body to function as intended, so we can respond to the challenges of everyday life. I love being stress free with no anxiety about anything or anyone. I have complete confidence that no matter what happens in my life, it happens in my best interest. I love feeling 20 years old and just beginning to live my childhood dreams. I am looking forward to the next 100 years and being in the moment every minute of every day. I refuse to let anyone ruin my day.

Using non-transdermal energy and noninvasive technology and the other things mentioned in this book, I have successfully overcome the symptoms of every disease and many aging processes. I have been successful not because I am smart enough to have figured out most of it myself, but because of my determination to succeed. Through prayer I have attracted the people into my life who have been kind enough to teach me what I needed to know when I needed it. I keep an open mind. I am eager to learn from everyone I meet or speak to on the phone, and I live in gratitude for each moment of life.

The energy I have been using and learning about has been of real benefit to me. Energy frequency can be targeted to any organ to enhance and activate particular systems. Once the energy is applied to the body, the frequency triggers communication specifically with the targeted organ and enhances the body's natural systems to assist it in rejuvenating.

Understanding how the body receives the energy: When you get a phone call, your phone emits an electromagnetic signal. The signal vibrates at the frequency associated with your cell phone number, which is how your phone "knows" the call is intended for it. Even though we can't see it, hear it or feel it, energy can affect every cell of all living things in a similar manner.

Energy can be either beneficial or detrimental (like cell phone EMR).Some research has shown that it may cause brain cancer. When magnetic energy is used properly, it can enhance cellular health.

The best results appear over time as your body assimilates bio-frequencies that maximize effects on the targeted system. Everybody is unique, so effects will vary for every person. The body's hydration level is key to optimizing the use of energy. It may be 2–3 months before you see the physical change, or as quickly as within minutes.

Our health is our choice. Live in love for all, and we will make the world a better place for everyone.

CHAPTER 21

Acidified Sodium Chlorite (MMS)

After 5 years of using it, my thoughts and experience, as it goes beyond health with its many benefits:

Most of my knowledge of acidified Sodium Chlorite (MMS) is from my friend Jim Humble. My stories are from personal experience and what I have written in my book is based on them. My opinion of the results I received are based on personal perceptions. I have done my best to state everything I have been able to accomplish in reversing my many health issues as it occurred, and attributed the results to what I felt gave them to me. Dr. Dean Bonlie gave me some specific corrections for a few things I had misunderstood, and I corrected them before my book went to print.

Just before I sent this in to be printed, I received an e-mail from Dr. Hesselink with his comments on what I had written. I did address some of the issues he pointed out. However, since some of what I feel I have experienced in reversing many of my health issues seems to contradict some of what Dr. Hesselink has stated, am posting his comments regarding chapter 21.

I know I have received all of the benefits I have written about, but it seems that I may be mistaken as to just how I received some of them. In other words, it was the combination of several things I was doing at the same time that allowed me to reverse a particular health issue, and not necessarily the use of acidified Sodium Chlorite (MMS), ozone, or magnetic therapy, that I received a benefit. In my effort to be helpful and to encourage others to search for their own solutions, please keep in mind that what worked for me may not work for you. I don't have the education to support everything I have done. I am just pointing out that I achieved many things that a lot of doctors said couldn't be done. It seems that, despite the disagreement of well-educated men like Dr. Hesselink, Jim Humble, and Dr. Hitt (along with a host of others that I have learned a great deal from), all of the knowledge I have gained from them has served me well. Over the past 20 years, it comes down to the fact that I have gone from feeling 90 years old to feeling better than I did when I was in my 20s. My book expresses my opinion about how I felt I accomplished that.

I will do my best to post Dr. Hesselink's comments in the appropriate place so that it will be easier for the reader to note a difference of opinion. Some of his comments were very difficult for me to follow, as some were contrary to what I felt I understood. I hope this difference of opinion will encourage readers to do their own research into why oxidative therapies may work. They have made such an important improvement in my life and have helped me come to believe that health is simple.

I have such great respect for Dr. Hesselink and Jim Humble that I want to thank them both for teaching me so much that has helped me with my health issues. I am not disagreeing with either of them about anything. It is quite possible that I have misunderstood some of what I thought they taught me. I am not trying to tell anyone what they should do; I am just telling what I have done that has worked so well for me. I am pointing out that what I have done may work for you. I feel that if anyone is determined to find out what they can do for themselves, the knowledge is here today, if the seeker is persistent. We all have the ability to make our health our choice.

Everyone has an opinion about most things, and I am not debating what is right and what is wrong. I want to leave this open for discussion in the hope that it will stimulate some others to do their own research on oxidative therapies. I know that one of my goals in writing this book is to encourage others to help with researching things that work for each of us. The use of MMS has really improved my life. It has improved my clarity of thought, saved my teeth, and improved my health. If it did nothing else but save my remaining teeth, that is a miracle to me, since one dentist assured me I would be toothless in 6 months. He thought I needed my remaining teeth pulled immediately in December 1996, but I have not lost a single tooth since brushing and flossing with acidified Sodium Chlorite (MMS).

With my new understanding of energy, it may be that just my belief that acidified Sodium Chlorite (MMS) would improve my health has provided the benefit. So many well-educated people dismiss the placebo effect; they see no value in it at all. They remain inside the box of whatever they were taught in school and continue to support double-blind studies. We all know that approximately one third of people who take a medication get well just because they think it will help. That alone is far better than the results of many drugs sold today. I would think that our government would want to spend some money on energy research to reduce our health care burden and national deficit.

I also realize that I may have been mistaken about how I received some of the benefits I wrote about in my heart chapter and my ozone chapter, as well. I have no doubt that I received the benefits, but I may have been mistaken as to the part oxidation played in my improving condition. I still believe it was an important part of reversing each condition I have written about, but some of the other things I was doing at the same time may have played a larger role than I felt they did at the time.

Editorial comments for chapter 21 per Dr. Thomas Hesselink, MD, January 30, 2012: I have placed Dr. Hesselink's comments into footnotes:

Mixing sodium chlorite with acid is what generates chlorine dioxide, which to be safely ingested must next be diluted in a big glass of water.

In addition to the many health benefits I have received from acidified Sodium Chlorite (MMS), it has given me clarity of thought that I haven't known since I was a young man. This has led to my spiritual awareness, which I couldn't imagine just a few years ago. This awakening motivated me to finish writing this book, so I could share what I have learned along with my personal experiences.

I have learned more about health and my spiritual awareness since taking Sodium Chlorite (MMS) over the past few years than I learned in my first 65 years of life. My clarity of thought has allowed me to explore my subconscious mind, seeking the answers that I feel are within us all. When I referred to my spirituality in this book, it was from my "then" point of view and little to do with religion. My views have evolved as I learn more and more, and I am still experiencing enlightenment. (I use "enlightenment" to mean knowledge and awareness that we are all eternal, spiritual beings: light-energy beings.) This is my story and these are my views only; they should not reflect on any other person mentioned in my book.

Jim Humble has been very patient with me and kind with his time to teach me a lot of what I know about health, along with dozens of doctors, chemists, and PhD's in various fields. Many other health care professionals have also taken time over the years to help me see what has become my picture of health; what I have learned has obviously worked well for me. All that these professionals have taught me, along with my personal experience with oxidative therapies, has supported most of what I have learned from Jim Humble about the benefits of oxidation.

One thing that has really stood out to me is that better-educated people, who are still seeking the truth, and who keep an open mind about what helps the body heal itself, are those who understand the benefits of oxidation quickest.

Sodium Chlorite (MMS) is quite likely to become the most important discovery in health in history. It can discriminate between pathogens and the friendly flora the body needs to maintain a healthy balance of microorganisms needed to digest food. Without this balance, we cannot properly extract the nutrients from what we eat. Dr. Sal D'Onofrio has stated that the digestive tract is the mother of our immune system. When it doesn't work properly, we can't maintain a healthy body.

Oxidants versus Antioxidants

Sodium Chlorite (MMS), when used properly in Jim Humble's protocol 1000, is an oxidant without equal and very little potential downside (if any). Some people experience nausea if they take too much at once, but in much smaller hourly dosages, 8 to 10 times a day, negative reactions are rare.

Nausea does occur when you take too much Sodium Chlorite (MMS) too fast, especially if you take it on an empty stomach. When this happens it usually goes away quickly by drinking water. If it persists, mash up a couple of vitamin C tablets, dissolve them in water, drink that with more water, and the nausea usually goes away in a short time.

I have felt that ozone (an oxidative therapy I used to help with my heart attacks) did help cleanse my circulatory system by oxidizing the plaque that caused the blockages leading to my three heart attacks. When I started using Sodium Chlorite (MMS), I felt it did the same thing, as I got a noticeable reduction in my blood pressure along with many other benefits I had previously received from the use of chelation therapy.

Dr. Thomas Hesselink:

Inflammation in the stomach immediately after ingestion is supposed to be treated by drinking more water until the nausea subsides.

Not sodium chlorite nor MMS nor chlorine dioxide dissolves away any plaque.

When nausea occurs, it is often referred to as a Herxheimer reaction. This represents the immune system ramping up inflam-

matory responses to kill pathogens; this does not overwhelm the lymph system with debris.

Oxidants support the immune system by oxidizing pathogens. Until I received the e-mail from Dr. Hesselink 1-30-12, I believed that Sodium Chlorite (MMS) discriminates in two ways.

At this moment I don't know what to think. I thought I had this book finished in August 2011, but 6 months later I am still editing it. I have had so many people kind enough to help me with this, and I want to make it as accurate as possible, but I can't put off publishing it forever. I will address the issue of how Sodium Chlorite (MMS) discriminates between pathogens in my newsletter and on my website when I can get additional accurate information on the subject.

I wrote this chapter before I received the e-mail from Dr. Hesselink and I am at a loss as to how to explain our differences of opinion, as I still feel that Sodium Chlorite (MMS) can discriminate between pathogens. I base this opinion on my ability to maintain a balance in my digestive flora. I no longer have any digestion issues I am aware of. I have no gas; I have normal bowel movements (at least 1 to normally 3 times a day). Prior to using Sodium Chlorite (MMS), I had a lot of indigestion issues that plagued me for more than 20 years.

1. First, I thought that nearly all pathogens were acidic and that Sodium Chlorite (MMS) attacked only acidic pathogens. I understand that pathogens thrive in an acidic environment.

   Dr. Thomas Hesselink: Generally speaking, harmful pathogens are not acidic—some produce acids, some produce gases, some produce alkalinity. It depends entirely on the metabolic process of the individual species.

   Even though this sounded plausible, I did not understand how it worked. I spoke with many doctors, chemists, and microbiologists who had different explanations and thoughts about the subject before I heard the statement below, which made more sense to me.

2. I have heard many doctors who lecture at trade shows state that many pathogens are anaerobic, meaning that they thrive in an oxygen-depleted environment and cannot live in an oxygen-rich environment. This leads me to believe that Sodium Chlorite (MMS) provides the oxygen that creates an inhospitable environment for pathogens.

   Dr. Thomas Hesselink – Most harmful pathogens are NOT anaerobic either; some are fully aerobic and require plenty of oxygen to grow. Others are microaerophyllic, preferring low oxygen levels; anaerobes must live under special circumstances where there is NO oxygen or they die from oxygen toxicity because their antioxidant protections are insufficient to cope with 20 percent oxygen exposure.

3. Dr. Hitt, MD, and microbiologist, explained that, in addition, all healthy cells create their own antioxidants to protect themselves from the effects of oxidation. The light came on in my head and Sodium Chlorite (MMS) and all forms of oxidation therapy made sense to me.

   By eliminating many types of pathogens, a lot of stress is naturally removed from the immune system, allowing it to be more effective and efficient even if the pathogens are not directly related to the health issue. Your immune system *can* be overloaded with work when you are sick; Sodium Chlorite (MMS) just contributes to the effort.

Jim Humble explained another way that Sodium Chlorite (MMS) discriminates using the cell's electrical charge in one of his classes. The explanation below is not verbatim, it is from my notes of Jim's class, but is my interpretation of what I believe he said.

Electrons hold everything together in the universe by forming a shell that holds it. *Protons* hold everything together; they attract electrons, which spin around atomic nuclei made of protons and neutrons. Extremely important, protons *cannot* be altered without serious manipulation (otherwise we could turn lead into gold). Electrons can be traded with ease; all you need is something with a stronger positive charge. This is how Sodium Chlorite (MMS) works: through electron exchange. Basically, Sodium Chlorite (MMS) oxidizes, or "rusts," cells by stealing electrons. Atoms are held together with energy created by electrons spinning around the nuclei. Neutrons are neutral atomic particles (in other words, they are not positive or negative). Each atom has its own vibrational frequency and individual characteristics. Electrons hold them together in molecules, which make up everything in the universe.

As Sodium Chlorite (MMS) gets near a pathogen molecule, it draws off the electrons; this is the oxidation process. As it draws them off, the pathogen is destroyed. Oxidation results in multiple holes in the surface of a pathogen. Once a pathogen loses its electrons, it just falls apart. Think about this as being similar to a cracker in water: eventually the cell turns into mush.

The measure of what a substance will and will not oxidize is called its oxidation-reduction potential (ORP).

Once activated, Sodium Chlorite (MMS) produces chlorine dioxide, and that's what destroys the pathogens. Oxidation only occurs when the particles being oxidized have an ORP less than the oxidant. Chlorine dioxide has a very low oxidation potential (it won't destroy much). It runs through the body without doing damage to healthy cells.

Dr. Thomas Hesselink: Chlorine dioxide kills certain organisms by destroying particular molecules on which they depend to survive. This process has nothing to do with aerobic or anaerobic. Most pathogens are neutral in electric charge if you add up all of the cations and anions, and this has nothing to do with oxidative therapies or antiseptic oxidants. Oxidants strip electrons off of the sensitive molecules they are reacting with and has nothing to do with the overall electrical charge of the organism.

Dr. Thomas Hesselink: MMS pulls electrons off of certain molecules inside or about the pathogen; it does not generally pull away electrons from just anything. MMS has a higher positive electron potential compared to the molecules it is able to oxidize. Voltages in electrochemistry pertain to relative comparisons among molecules and which direction the electrons will tend to migrate.

Other oxidants destroy pathogens as well

Ozone is one of the most powerful oxidizers I am aware of and is used very successfully for health issues in many countries around the world. It has an ORP of 2.7 millivolts and will destroy anything that can be oxidized in the body with an ORP of less than 2.7. Jim Humble said that ozone works very well, but it does not get deep enough into the tissues. Therefore, it can destroy some friendly flora and cause damage to healthy cells, as well as pathogens. This is because many of our friendly flora fall in the range of an ORP of .95 to 2.7. Since Sodium Chlorite (MMS) is at .95 and ozone is at 2.7, Sodium Chlorite (MMS) is a better choice as most pathogens are .9 and below. In addition, ozone's half-life is very short and quickly loses its benefit.

Dr. Thomas Hesselink: Chlorine dioxide is weaker than ozone, but certainly not weak, as 0.95 volts is still pretty hefty for an oxidant in electrochemistry. The problem with ozone has little to do with depth and everything to do with reactivity. Ozone reacts with so many different molecules that it readily gets used up.

Dr. Thomas Hesselink: Chlorine dioxide is more selective, and by serendipity hits special molecules that pathogens must have to thrive. Ozone practices much less discrimination.

Another oxidizer, hydrogen peroxide, is available in health food stores and drug stores, most commonly at a 3 percent solution. As far as I know, 30–35 percent food grade is the strongest concentration available and is the one most commonly used by health care practitioners and those looking for ways to help themselves when medication does not.

Hydrogen peroxide has an ORP of 1.8 millivolts. I used it until it created a very bad taste in my mouth. Within 2 weeks of stopping, that bad taste cleared up. That was the only downside I noticed, but I have talked to several microbiologists, chemists, and doctors who have all warned me about the harmful side effects of using too much.

I noticed that the 35 percent food grade was not available for a very long time. Many years later, it reappeared as something that was going to save humankind. The *One Minute Cancer Cure* is about hydrogen peroxide. I have heard many good things about hydrogen peroxide and personally experienced some impressive benefits. I gargled with it on and off since the 1940s and 1950s to control tonsillitis, which reoccurs several times every winter with great results. However, after meeting Jim Humble and understanding Sodium Chlorite (MMS), I quickly realized that the latter has far less potential downside.

> *Dr. Thomas Hesselink: Hydrogen peroxide is even more restricted and selective, despite its voltage compared to other molecules.* H_2O_2 *is much more slowly reactive than chlorine dioxide. I recommend against 35 percent peroxide because too many people get hurt mishandling it.*

Oxygen has an ORP of 1.3 millivolts. Even oxygen destroys some of the friendly flora along with other important cellular life in the body.

Chlorine dioxide has an oxidation potential of 0.95 millivolts. There are no healthy cells or friendly flora that I know of that can be negatively affected by 0.95 millivolts. The only things it can affect are things that come into the body, such as pathogens, heavy metals, and poisons. I believe that most, if not all, have a charge of less than 0.95; this seems to be the biggest reason that Sodium Chlorite (MMS) discriminates.

Jim is a very smart man, and I have a great deal of respect for him and his research. I don't have the educational background to know for sure that it is 100 percent correct, but I do believe that Jim does. It helps me to understand some of the science of why Sodium Chlorite (MMS) is the most important health product I have ever run across, because I have seen the results of using it. I think he is truly a great humanitarian. I have no doubt that his work will save millions of lives throughout the world.

Dr. Thomas Hesselink: Jim Humble is smart, but that is not why MMS works. MMS works because chlorine dioxide (ClO_2) specifically targets sensitive molecules in pathogens. He was astute to observe this benefit firstly in malaria and later in other diseases. It is more rapid acting than hydrogen peroxide (H_2O_2) or oxygen (O_2). It is more selective than ozone (O_3), and it is way, way safer than elemental chlorine (Cl_2) or sodium hypochlorite (NaClO).

Antioxidants protect the body's cells from potential damage by free radicals in the body. The body needs a balance of everything to maintain a stable environment. Whether it is yin and yang, pH, body temperature, or oxidants and antioxidants, balance is important to maintain an internal environment that is conducive to the synergy needed for optimal health.

Dr. Thomas Hesselink:– I agree that the body has—and carefully controls at all times, to the best of its ability—a careful balance between oxidants and antioxidants. Antioxidants support healing and growth; oxidants destroy sensitive pathogens and stimulate immune reactivity.

The oxygen in the air we breathe, along with ozone, hydrogen peroxide, and Sodium Chlorite (MMS), can all cause oxidation. Oxidation acts like free radicals and may cause some cellular damage, and antioxidants play an important part in its prevention and/or repair. Many doctors and researchers have said, "Because oxidants and antioxidants do opposite things, they would naturally neutralize each other." That sounded logical, and I believed it to be true for many years.

The manufacturers of ASEA, a relatively new product, have found a way to stabilize 8 oxidants and 8 antioxidants that all retain their attributes while mixed in a solution, for over a year and a half. When I learned this, the light came on; I realized that most of the old thinking had to be wrong.

Many well-educated, well-meaning people are stuck in a box with what they were taught, and believe it to be right. I believe my advantage has been my lack of formal education, which has helped me to remain outside the box and open to receiving all points of view. Discussing all subjects with everyone I encounter is exciting to me, whether we agree or not. We can learn from everyone as long as we keep an open mind.

It now makes sense to me that if we step up our intake of oxidants, we should increase the intake of antioxidants too. Even though I have never noticed any benefit from taking antioxidants, I have received many incredible benefits from oxidants. I now believe there should be a balance between them. I no longer believe that they neutralize each other when there is an adequate separation of time between taking them. There may not even be a need for a separation in time at all, but I will leave that up to the experts who want to make health seem complicated to prove one way or the other.

Since so little research has been done on the need to balance oxidants and antioxidants, I don't believe anyone can say for sure how much of either we should take or how close together we can take them. One of the most important reasons I would like to have my book as widely disseminated as possible is to encourage scientists and researchers to take my stories of the anecdotal benefits of oxidation and find the answers that will help improve our world's health.

As I noted in Chapter 2, one of the first benefits I noticed using Sodium Chlorite (MMS) was in my eyesight. After 15 drops both morning and night for about 6 weeks, I noticed a big benefit to both my eyesight and my short-term memory. It was very exciting to think it had only cost me $20 this time instead of $1000 worth of IV chelation. 5 years later, I still maintain these benefits.

On my weekly conference calls and on phone calls I receive every day, I have spoken to thousands of people with incredible stories to share about the benefits of Sodium Chlorite (MMS). I believe there is no other product that can come close to its potential to help the body heal itself.

It is important to point out that a lot of what I have learned about the benefits of oxidants and Sodium Chlorite (MMS) has been through many doctors and health care professionals who have the educational background to understand the science behind it and why it works so well.

The few people who have looked for ways to discredit Sodium Chlorite (MMS) have not had the personal experience that I have, and have not seen its benefits for many others firsthand. It is a shame that a few people look for the negative and spread fear about anything they haven't used for whatever their reasons may be. Everything in life needs balance, just as there are good and evil. If there were no "dark" side with its own agenda to rule over the world, "light" workers would have no place to shine.

Most of us have heard this verse from the Bible: "Seek and ye shall find." Most of us are stuck in the middle between the light workers and the dark agenda as we are influenced by so many misinterpretations of the Bible, the Koran, and hundreds of other religious writings. Most of us tend to live our lives in the gray area between light and dark—for many, that means in the fog. When we have many health problems, we often can't think rationally, since our thoughts are about survival and eliminating the pain that often accompany disease.

I have never felt better in my entire life than I do today, and I owe much of it to Jim Humble and Sodium Chlorite (MMS). I highly recommend Jim's book in order to fully understand the science behind it. You can get a copy at www.jimhumble.biz. Another valuable resource for a better understanding of all forms of oxidative therapies is Dr. Tom Hesselink's website, http://bioredox.mysite.com. He has been very helpful; calling me several times to let me know there was something on my website that was not correct. He is one of the many doctors who have added a great deal to my understanding of oxidative therapies.

Robert Young, Gaston Naessens, and Royal Raymond Rife, who are all world-renowned microbiologists, have proven beyond a doubt that health is dependent on our internal environment.

Meeting Jim Humble, February 2006, Hermosillo, Mexico

I flew from Las Vegas to Hermosillo to spend some time with my friend, Ed, at his home in Kino Bay, Sonora, Mexico. Because communications there at the time were poor, I couldn't use my cell phone, so he did not know what time I would arrive, just the day. He said to call him from a pay phone when I arrived at the airport, and he would come pick me up.

Fortunately, when I arrived and called Ed, he had just spoken to Jim Humble on the telephone and Jim was only a few minutes away from the airport. Since Jim had been staying at Ed's and was on his way there anyway, we arranged for Jim to give me a ride.

I asked, "How will I know what to look for and how will I recognize Jim?" Ed said, "Don't worry; you will have no problem recognizing him; he looks just like an old prospector with a funny hat, like you see in the movies. He really stands out." I was a little apprehensive with such a vague description, but Ed was right. Before long, here was an old guy with a hat that looked like something that Indiana Jones wore. But there was no doubt in my mind of who he was.

Jim was very friendly, polite, and informative about the area and what Kino Bay was like. I hadn't been to Kino Bay since 1964. There was not much there at all then. I found Jim to be extremely intelligent and fascinating with all the stories about his discovery of Sodium Chlorite (MMS). He was driven to share the success he had experienced using this product.

Over the next 3 months, I found Jim to be a real humanitarian. He believed in the product and couldn't keep from giving it to everyone in need that we came across. Here he was, living off of his Social Security and just barely getting by financially, yet giving away this lifesaving product rather than selling it. I asked him one day, "Don't you think you could be more of a benefit to more people by selling Sodium Chlorite (MMS) to those who can afford it? Then you could afford to give more to those who can't."

He replied, "Yes, but the law won't allow me to do both!" He said, "You cannot sell and tell; that is the law in the United States, and I feel that getting my book out to the world is far more important than trying to make a few dollars from selling the product."

I was really moved by his passion that Sodium Chlorite (MMS) could make a difference in the world. By this time in our friendship, I had already experienced some very noticeable benefits from using it myself, and I was starting to understand why he was so driven to make everyone aware of its potential to make the world a better place for all. I realized then that Jim might be the answer to my prayers for the opportunity to do just that. I had really wanted to find a way to set an example for my children, to help them see that we are not on earth to indulge ourselves in a meaningless life, but to benefit one another. Five years later, I realize my prayers were answered when I met Jim. For years now, I had asked for the opportunity to give my life meaning and purpose and to be a benefit to others. Now, seldom a day goes by when someone doesn't call just to thank me for helping them with Sodium Chlorite (MMS).

After about 6 weeks, I was learning so much from Ed and Jim that I wasn't about to leave. It was like having my own personal professors, both eager to teach me. Between them, they were able to answer just about any question about health and nearly any other subject I had an interest in. The three months we lived together were among the most memorable times of my life; this was just the beginning of my education. What I learned helped me to understand what was taking place with my own health improvements. I was able to picture just how simple health can be as I lived it and understood what was happening in my body, mind, and soul.

It is not that Jim and Ed always agreed on everything or that I accepted everything they so persistently taught, but we all kept open minds. Our minds gave us the truth that made us all better prepared to fulfill our own purposes in life. I believe we all learned from one another; I far more than either of them. For me, it was an experience of a lifetime. I felt we all parted with a common goal of doing what we could to help the world become a better place. In October 2011, Jim told me that what he has been doing is not fun; it is a lot of hard work. He does it because it is the right thing to do for the sake of humanity. I feel the same way as he does and agree with his saying, "Always do what is right; do the right thing." It comes to mind often when I am trying to decide what direction I should go in my effort to be of service: how can I be of most benefit to others?

I often recall having lunch with Christopher Hegarty, a former Catholic bishop and one of the most memorable men I have ever met. Our lunch lasted from 11:00 a.m. until almost dark. He told me basically the same thing as Jim Humble. "When the struggles of life seem to be overwhelming and you don't know which way to turn, life becomes simple when you choose to do the right thing." He went on to say that, in his last prayer of the day, he always asks God to please send him someone that he may help each day. That is our reason for living: to learn to live in love for one another and to help make the world a better place for us all.

This story is important to me because both men, I believe, have a similar belief in their effort to be a benefit to humanity. I feel they both have earned the right to be proud of their contributions and the right to claim the title of bishop, even though their religious beliefs are different. They both do what they feel is right for them and for the benefit of others.

At the end of March 2007, the most noticeable benefits I had realized in my first 6 weeks on Sodium Chlorite (MMS) were:

1. My gums had stopped bleeding when I brushed my teeth in just 4 days.
2. My teeth were noticeably much tighter. I was no longer concerned about losing my remaining teeth as this was working so well.
3. I had a noticeable improvement in my short-term memory.
4. I had a noticeable improvement in my attention span. (I no longer had many "senior moments", jumping from subject to subject and not remaining focused on anything.)
5. I had a noticeable improvement in my eyesight.
6. There was a major improvement in my overall pain level.
7. I had a noticeable improvement in my energy level.

Two years later, I had zero plaque on my teeth, even though I hadn't had them cleaned in three years. It has been five years now, and I have not lost a tooth. I was told I was six months away from being toothless about the time I started using MMS.

At this point, Jim had been recommending that users activate each drop of 28 percent Sodium Chlorite (MMS) solution with two drops of apple cider vinegar. After three minutes, this produced chlorine dioxide, which was added to a few ounces of water and drinking it within a few minutes.

In April 2007, I took Jim Humble and Ed to see Dr. William Hitt and Dr. John Humiston. All four spent many hours teaching me a lot of what I know. Dr. Hitt realized that Sodium Chlorite (MMS) is an oxidant that acted similarly to ozone, so he was very interested in learning more about it. Dr. Humiston joined in quickly. Jim left them one of his books and a bottle of Sodium Chlorite (MMS). In May, the Hitt Center called to ask for 30 more bottles, as soon as I could get them there. I was so excited that I left the next day and drove 14 hours to deliver it.

Jim could not sell Sodium Chlorite (MMS). At that time, the only person in the world who did was Kenneth Richardson in Canada. So I became its first distributor in the United States. Kenneth very helpfully explained how to safely package and ship the product. I can't thank him enough for all of his help.

Not long afterward, Dr. Humiston called me and said that the blood analysis on his patients showed that fungus was adapting to the environment created by the Sodium Chlorite (MMS). He suggested using lemon or lime juice instead of vinegar, because vinegar is a fermented substance that feeds fungus, making it harder to get rid of.

He pointed out that most of Jim's experience had been with malaria. Since only two doses were needed to handle the parasite that caused that disease, there was no opportunity for fungus to adapt (though fungus isn't related to malaria anyway); it is understandable that Jim was never aware of this problem before.

I relayed this information to Jim, and he made the correction. He called me a few months later to tell me he was getting even better results activating with citric acid. I was reluctant to change, as I had just corrected all my printed material, and I couldn't even find a place to buy citric acid at that time. I finally ordered it through Wal-Mart Pharmacy at a cost of $24 for 1 pound plus tax.

I found it to be so much more convenient, and it did seem to work better. Once I started to make it in a 50 percent solution, the activation time dropped from 3 minutes to 30 seconds. It was now more convenient and more affordable for everyone.

Dr. Thomas Hesselink: Once I became familiar with the chemistry of the oxides of chlorine as a class of inorganic compounds, I determined that any edible and non-reductive acid that can bring the pH down close to 2.0 should work. Citric acid is preferred because it can be transported as a dry powder and easily produces a strongly acidic solution. Tartaric acid or succinic acid or isocitric would have been fine, but most non-chemists are familiar with citric acid as this is so commonly found in citrus fruit and is worldwide as a commonly used food additive. Remind people not to load up on antioxidants such as vitamin C, cysteine, or glutathione before an oxidative therapy or the medicinal oxidants will be destroyed before they can do their job.

I am not dogmatic about this, but 20 percent sodium chlorite (made from 25 percent technical grade) mixed with 10 percent citric acid in equal volumes works fine.

I feel that I have more experience than anyone in the world using Sodium Chlorite (MMS) with the exception of Jim Humble himself. I have used it longer and more successfully than anyone else I am aware of. I have talked to thousands about it, and only a few have not seen any benefit. When Jim started giving his classes in the Dominican Republic, he called me and invited me to come down. I was reluctant at first, because I had so many things going on at that time. I always enjoy spending time with Jim, but I really didn't expect to learn very much more from him, as I felt he had already taught me all he knew.

I went to Jim's class in June 2010 and was pleasantly surprised by how much more Jim had learned from three-plus more years of research. I took 70 pages of notes the first week, then went to Haiti and took many more. I have traveled much of the world and have seen many things, but this was the most unforgettable trip I have ever made.

Jim offered far more than a class about health. It was a life-changing experience. There was not one person attending who was not exceptional. I admired and respected every one of them.

I think the most important thing that I learned in Jim's classes is his protocol 1000, which has the potential to help the body to heal itself of most health issues.

Mixing sodium chlorite with acid is what generates chlorine dioxide, which to be safely ingested must next be diluted in a glass of water with a minimum of 1 once of water to each drop of acidified Sodium Chlorite (MMS).

The new protocol 1000 is to take 1 drop of activated Sodium Chlorite (MMS) each hour to start with, and then work up to 3 drops every hour for 8 hours in a row for 21 days.

All references are made to "a drop" of activated Sodium Chlorite (MMS). It is best to use 1 drop of 50 percent citric acid to 1 drop of Sodium Chlorite (MMS). If you are going to ingest it, remember "1-1-1:"

- 1 drop of Sodium Chlorite (MMS)
- 1 drop of Citric Acid
- 1 ounce of water *30 seconds later.*

The best way to mix this is to use a glass bottle. I am sure you can still find a 1-quart glass bottle (32 ounces). Fill it with reverse osmosis-filtered or distilled water.

A. Use a clean, dry glass and add 32 drops of Sodium Chlorite (MMS).

B. Add 32 drops of citric acid (50 percent solution). Swish it around to make sure it is all mixed well and let sit for 30 seconds.

C. Take your quart bottle of water and pour a few ounces of it into the glass, then pour it all back into the bottle and put the cap on fairly tightly. This solution will stay activated for a week or more at room temperature (longer in the refrigerator).

D. On the first day, drink 1 ounce every hour. You can dilute it with more water if you like. Jim has some suggestions if you feel the need to hide the taste. Many people find that essential oil of peppermint works very well.

E. Providing there are no adverse effects the first day (such as nausea, or diarrhea), move up the number of drops, 8 times per day as directed below.

F. On the second day, take 2 ounces of the solution—2 drops of the active Sodium Chlorite (MMS)—each hour, 8 times per day, if you have no adverse effects.

G. On the third day, take 3 drops each hour. Stay at that dose 8 times a day for 21 days. At the first sign of nausea, drop back to the last dose that you could handle with no ill effects.

The most common side effect is nausea, in some cases diarrhea; a few people get headaches. If you notice any other side effect you feel may be related, you should reduce the number of drops, but try not to stop altogether. A fluctuating internal environment will contribute to the adaptation of fungus to the environment created by the Sodium Chlorite (MMS).

A lot of people think that if a little Sodium Chlorite (MMS) is good, a lot is better. I've heard people say, "I can take a little bit of sickness; I'll just increase the dosages and get well quicker." ***But that's not the way to do it***. If you allow yourself to get sick from using too much, it reduces the effectiveness of the Sodium Chlorite (MMS) and increases the healing time. Nausea and diarrhea use up the energy you need to heal. Don't allow the Sodium Chlorite (MMS) to make you feel worse. It's a good indicator of the condition of your body at first, but be sure to back off by 1 drop each hour if you become nauseated. In other words, if you are doing a 3-drop dose and you experience nausea or diarrhea, you should reduce to a 2-drop dose. If you are still feeling sick, reduce to a 1-drop dose.

I have spoken with a few people who started with only a teaspoon of the prepared solution an hour; this equals just 1/6 of a drop. But they were persistent; and within a few weeks, they were up to 3 drops an hour.

Another person, after trying many ways to take Sodium Chlorite (MMS), felt they may have an allergy to citric acid. They opted to use lemon juice and were able to take it without any ill effects at all.

From my notes taken in Jim Humble's class, Jim says he has been getting about the same results taking Sodium Chlorite (MMS) as an enema, as he is when taking it as an IV. Although it is inconvenient, it is a very good way to maximize the potential benefit without any ill effects.

I have used it in this manner by using 8 activated drops in 16 oz. of warm water and inserting just 8 oz., holding it for 10 to 15 minutes. Then expelling and doing it a second time. I better explained this in chapter 20.

> *Dr. Thomas Hesselink: I would not trust people to dilute solutions appropriately if you are going to suggest enemas. Drinking is self-limited (due to the smell, the nausea); enemas could cause damage before this is sensed subjectively. Go ahead and write something like that in, but let me review it because I think artery disease has so many different causes that it is inappropriate to look to any one remedy to treat it.*

This new protocol is good for most illnesses. If you come across an illness that you don't know about, or you are not sure what to do about treating it, you should consider starting with Jim's protocol 1000. Jim lists many protocols for using Sodium Chlorite

(MMS) in his book. He teaches them in his monthly classes. They were the best education I ever got for addressing my own health issues.

Dr. Thomas Hesselink: Jim definitely did all of us and many others an honorable favor by sharing his experiences.

Disclaimer: I am not an expert on anything; I am a student of health and life, an observer who documents what is. As my education continues to progress, I see and learn more about the truth of the simplicity of health, and the more enjoyable life becomes. I am driven by a desire to learn anything and everything I can that will help me with my many health issues, and I know we will all have many more throughout our lives. Why not take the opportunity to learn all we can to minimize negative effects when they do occur? My desire is to be open to learn from everyone who is willing to share their knowledge with me.

The information in my book has allowed me to be very successful in restoring my own health. I can't tell you how to treat yourself or anyone else. I can tell you about my personal experiences, which I have studied and researched while treating my own health issues. I am making no medical claims; I am just making observations of results I have had. I hope you see the value of my efforts and my desire to give you ideas about what to try if you choose to accept responsibility for your own health, while you do your own research.

Please join me as a fellow researcher in the effort to learn how to achieve and maintain our own health and help others do the same, through our own education and life's experiences. I believe the technology is here today to eliminate all disease. It is up to us, as freethinking people, to share knowledge with each other and allow everyone to live in optimum health. I believe the information will benefit each of us, our country, and all of humanity.

My Purpose In Life

I wrote the above in June of 2007 when I first understood just how simple health can be. I have felt I had found my purpose in life before. As I continue to learn more, my purpose changes as I see new and better ways I can be of service to humanity.

I believe my purpose is to share all that I have learned that makes health seem so simple to me now. My hope and expectation is that everyone who has the desire to learn what we can do to make our health our choice will be able to reverse their health issues and aging process, as I have successfully done. I firmly believe *Your Health is Your Choice*—as is your life!

I hope to inspire everyone to read what I have been able to accomplish over the past 20 years, since retiring from the fire department. I went from feeling 90 years old then to feeling 20 today. When I heard that nearly all disease comes from a pathogen or environmental toxin, it made sense. I was already aware that disease evolved depending on the weakness of our individual DNA. The light came on in my head and health became simple.

I then realized I had to become a part of taking Jim's work to the world. It became a compulsion. I felt that God had blessed me with this knowledge and the ability to reverse all of my health issues, along with my aging process, and it is my obligation to share it with the world.

I finally realized that the reason for living is for the opportunity to change ourselves. We are all a part of our world's consciousness; as we become aware of this and change our way of thinking to, and desire to, live our lives for the benefit of one another and the betterment of humanity, the world will just naturally respond.

This is my story, I see everyone as a spiritual being, a part of a unified energy field, and I respect everyone's religious beliefs. I have attempted not to express any religious views. My thoughts of my spiritual awareness are mine alone and are not meant to reflect on anyone other than myself. I am still seeking enlightenment that will lead me to a better understanding of what I can do to help make the world a better place for us all.

God bless us all.

"May your book be a success!"

—Doc Tom Hesselink, http://bioredox.mysite.com

Chapter 22

Future Projects and Thoughts from the Author

My plan for the future is to continue to write about the new and exciting things that I learn every day that are changing my life and our world. I am learning about quantum physics and realizing we are all a part of a quantum energy field. We are all a part of this paradigm shift, like it or not and it is happening now. My vision is of a world without sickness, disease, pain, and suffering; a world filled with the joy of living in love for one another. I believe that together we can achieve this, as we are all one with God and one with every other person on this earth. Frankly, I believe, we are even as one with others in faraway solar systems. We are all part of the same unified energy field, and each of us is capable of manifesting our wants, needs, and desires.

I did not just wake up with this concept one morning; this is what I have come to believe through my life's experiences. It has been a learning process over many years. As I look back over my life, the words of wisdom from many sources come flooding back into my consciousness. I am open to learn from everyone I meet and often have the opportunity to share information with people from little children to well-educated doctors, scientists, and scholars.

Writing has been a very important part of my learning process. It is my desire that it become a benefit to you as well. You see, I learn far more about a new subject by *writing* about what learn when I am learning it. In this way, I can continue to add to each concept, because with time, I am able to see more of the picture of life, our health, and our purpose for living. I see life as a puzzle, and as we age, we learn more about it. Realizing that I am a visual person, I need to "see" the picture of life. Writing my life's experiences helps me to learn and to remember more of the details as I continue to see more of the puzzle's picture through life lessons. It just makes it easier to put the rest of the puzzle together.

The more open we are to learning from one another, the more benefit we offer to others, our families, and our loved ones. This can give us the satisfaction of living our lives with meaning and purpose, once we understand that we have helped to make the world a better place.

Energy Medicine: I feel that what I am manifesting will continue to bring many more people into my life who will teach me what I need to know to fulfill my dream. My dream and my prayer is to be of service to humanity. I have prayed for many years for the opportunity to help make the world a better place for us all. I have no doubt that I will learn a lot more about energy medicine. I am certain it is the future of our health and our very existence.

We are energy beings! We are 99.9999 percent space, held together with the energy produced by our bodies, and yet most of us have no concept of how this works. I mentioned that I learned this in 1954, in Mr. Jeff's 7th-grade science class. I thought he was crazy. It has taken me well over 50 years to understand what he was explaining to us. Energy is like the air we breathe. We cannot see it, smell it, feel it, taste it, or touch it, but we know it is there and we know it is vital to life. The earth's magnetic energy is just as important to life as the air we breathe. Few of us have any understanding of this vital necessity, which supports life as we know it, much less this energy's ability to accelerate our healing process.

Physicians who use energy include Dr. Steven Daniel, Dr. Sal D'Onofrio, Dr. Howard Hagglund, Dr. John Humiston, and Dr. Bradley Nelson. They are my friends and have been my guests on my conference calls every Tuesday night. There are many others who are also using energy to help us heal ourselves. Each of these physicians has so much information to contribute to our knowledge of life and our health. Once we understand what they have to share with us, life will become much more pleasant as we learn to manifest. Everyone is invited to become a part of our phone family by signing up for our club at www.DrHealthClub.com, or look on line for www.YourHealthIsYourChoice.org.

It has taken me most of my life to understand what I was taught in Sunday school back in the early 1940s, when I first heard that Jesus Christ said, "the least among you can do all that I have done, and even greater things." I now realize we really do have this ability within us. I have experienced a spontaneous healing of my stage 4, untreatable liver cirrhosis. I have mentioned how I was diagnosed in June of 2009 and was told that a liver transplant was my only hope; 3 months later, it was healed with energy—in 1 ½ hours!

I wish to share this type of information as I continue to learn how this was possible. Health is simple, as is anything we understand. Some time ago, Dr. Hitt and Dr. Humiston explained that only the body can heal itself and that we simply need to give it a chance. They explained that the underlying cause of most disease is some form of pathogen or environmental toxin. Disease evolves into different types of health issues depending on the relative weakness of our individual DNA. In most cases, the same treatment will eliminate or at least help with most health issues. It is important to understand that we need a balance of oxidants and anti-oxidants.

Through my understanding of and experience with ozone, and later with Sodium Chlorite (MMS), I realized that oxidation addressed most health issues, as most pathogens and many environmental toxins cannot survive in the internal environment enriched by oxidants. That was when I realized that health is simple and affordable to most of us.

Health Club: I am in the process of creating an interactive health club that is unlike what most of us understand a health club to be (that is, one that focuses on exercise and fitness). I want to create this club for members to share information on a blog. The site, www.DrHealthClub.com, is already under construction. It will offer free membership and full access to a large forum about health and wellness. It will also offer special discounts on health and wellness products from manufacturers producing only the best of the best—quality products endorsed by the club for the benefit of its members. I will host questions, provide answers, and include testimonials from members, all with the participation of several of my friends who are experts in the health field.

Health Club members will receive updates on new research and have free access to my book updates, along with pictures I have taken to help you better understand what I write.

If you would like to become a member, please e-mail info@yourhealthisyourchoice.org.

Conference Calls: For the past 3 years now, I have been hosting free conference calls every Tuesday from 5:45 p.m. to 8:00 p.m. (PST).

I have had many remarkable guests on these calls, all with their own unique insights on health. They all possess pieces of the puzzle of life and health. As host of these calls, I have received the opportunity to learn from many spiritually guided people who are caring enough to share their knowledge and experiences, and callers have had the opportunity to ask questions and get answers from these experts. For those who care to participate and have the desire to learn, it is like having access to free consultations with a health care provider.

Conference Call Information: You can listen and ask questions live. For information on how to take advantage of this opportunity, please visit www.YourHealthisYourChoice.org or www.DrHealthClub.com.

You may listen to past calls and watch videos on the websites by going to the Media Archives at each one as well.

I am continually seeking new ways to achieve both mental and physical longevity; after all, we are whole beings: "body, mind, and soul."

My continuing mission is to be my own guinea pig, trying all that I can in my effort to become all that I can be. At this moment, I feel 20 years old. While the condition of my cellular structure is currently closer to my true age, I do expect that to change. I am right now evaluating a product and some energy techniques that I expect will allow my DNA to replicate as it did when I was very young. I will write about what I learn and will spread what I discover around the planet, as well as discuss the information on my calls.

I will be posting information from experts such as Dr. Mathias Rath, Dr. Mercola, Dr. Oz, Jim Humble, and other medical professionals who all have visions that can change the world with their knowledge and the use of a few products not produced by pharmaceutical companies.

I encourage all of my readers to write their own stories, if for no other reason than to help themselves with their own health issues—but doing so may help others as well. I hope many will write their own honest reviews of my book and post them on my blog and elsewhere. I feel that my message of hope will benefit many, so please help me in spreading the word**. Only we can make a difference in our lives, our health, and our world.**

As we connect with and bring together spiritually guided people from around the world, we can learn from one another how to change ourselves and the world. We have the capability to change the vibrational frequency of the earth. A paradigm shift is taking place at this time. This shift will allow us all to transcend the three-dimensional world that we now know; it is taking us into a higher dimension. We are all a part of this transformation, whether we consciously contribute to it or not. However, it is our choice whether to change ourselves and help make earth a better place for everyone.

My Vision: I hope that many readers will become ambassadors for the message that I have attempted to make clear in my book. If you are sick, and modern allopathic doctors who prescribe drugs have left you little to no hope...*Do not despair!* Many alternative doctors and other individuals want to help. There are so many others, not just doctors, who possess pieces of the puzzle of life and health. They understand that new scientific knowledge and the latest in healing techniques, which have been suppressed, will help!

We can improve our lives, create better health, and extend our longevity once we understand and believe in our ability to change. If a retired firefighter like me can do it, you can do it too!

Please help me spread the word that our lives and our health depend on our determination to do what needs to be done to make our life and our health our choice.

As a young child, I really struggled with reading and writing because I was dyslexic. However, through determination, I have been able to succeed in reversing all of my many health issues. I believe it is within everyone's ability to do the same once they understand my experiences and what I have accomplished by doing my own research!

It is my wish that you will share my book with others in the hope that it will encourage people from around the world. Don't give up on your life or your health. We all have the ability to help ourselves and the ones we love.

Only you can change your life and your health, as only your body can heal itself.

That makes *Your Health Your Choice*!

Thank you for taking the time to read my book. I invite you to join with me in my future projects. I hope you will share your life's experiences with us, because we all have knowledge and experiences that can help each other. We should aspire to support each other on this journey through life. Keep in mind that we all have this in common: we either have a health issue, or we will soon have one.

As I continue to learn about the new research from those I connect with, I will keep you posted. I hope you will take the time to help us bring our world into harmony, through the vibration of love for all.

Please become an active part of this concept, with the goal of bringing spiritually guided people together to share our lives and our stories. Please add your positive energy to our unified energy field by joining the club at www.DrHealthClub.com.

You can keep up with our progress by monitoring the website www.YourHealthisYourChoice.org. Your Health is Your Choice.

Live in Love and Light,
Dennis Richard

If you send me a copy of what you write and allow me to add you to my database, I will keep you posted on my latest research as I continue to discover new information that will help us all become connected and one with each other while allowing us to improve our life and our health.

Please send your e-mail to info@yourhealthisyourchoice.org.

NOTE: I no longer sell MMS or Sodium Chlorite, but I still use it. I do recommend that everyone consider using it. We all have viral loads, fungal loads, and other pathogens that break down our immune systems. Anything we can do to reduce these will help support the immune system that helps the body heal itself.

While writing my book, I have become aware of a project to enact a medical freedom of choice bill that needs to be in all state constitutions. It is called the "Dr. Benjamin Rush Amendment," named after one of the major leaders of the American Revolution and signer of the Declaration of Independence.

Dr. Rush commented during the debate on the Bill of Rights: that "medical freedom of choice and practice should be protected by the constitution or the day would come when we lose that freedom to government tyranny and a conspiracy of doctors to control medicine."

I have seen the FDA abuse their authority with regulations governing our freedom to buy and use the products we need to treat ourselves, so I am asking everyone to work together to help support the Rush Amendment. Jack Phillips, who is the author of the Rush Amendment, proves our current situation with over 100 years of evidence in his book, *Suppressed Medical Science*. The Dr. Rush Amendment website is www.rush2013.com.

I know of no other plan of action to counteract the tyranny we face today. We all need to get politically active and work at local and state levels to implement this bill to protect our health freedom.

The admonition below is attributed to Dr. Benjamin Rush, signer of the Declaration of Independence, during the time of the 1787–1791 Constitutional Convention.

"The Constitution of this Republic should make special provision for medical freedom. To restrict the art of healing to one class will constitute the Bastille of medical science. All such laws are un-American and despotic...Unless we put medical freedom into the Constitution; the time will come when medicine will organize into an undercover dictatorship and force people, who wish doctors and treatments of their own choice, to submit to only what the dictating outfit offers. The Constitution of the Republic should make a Special provision for medical freedoms as well as religious freedom."

Please help me with the distribution of my book by tearing off the information below and giving it to a friend.

Dennis Richard has posted videos that will help you better understand some of the things discussed in *Your Health Is Your Choice*. To view them, go to:

www.YourHealthisYourChoice.org / www.DrHealth.com / www.DRhealthclub.com

Or go to **www.youtube.com and search for DennisRichard-books and MMSdr1**

Please help me with the distribution of my book by tearing off the information below and giving it to a friend.

Dennis Richard has posted videos that will help you better understand some of the things discussed in *Your Health Is Your Choice*. To view them, go to:

www.YourHealthisYourChoice.org / www.DrHealth.com / www.DRhealthclub.com

Or go to **www.youtube.com and search for DennisRichard-books and MMSdr1**

Please help me with the distribution of my book by tearing off the information below and giving it to a friend.

Dennis Richard has posted videos that will help you better understand some of the things discussed in *Your Health Is Your Choice*. To view them, go to:

www.YourHealthisYourChoice.org / www.DrHealth.com / www.DRhealthclub.com

Or go to **www.youtube.com and search for DennisRichard-books and MMSdr1**

Please help me with the distribution of my book by tearing off the information below and giving it to a friend.

Dennis Richard has posted videos that will help you better understand some of the things discussed in *Your Health Is Your Choice*. To view them, go to:

www.YourHealthisYourChoice.org / www.DrHealth.com / www.DRhealthclub.com

Or go to **www.youtube.com and search for DennisRichard-books and MMSdr1**

Please help me with the distribution of my book by tearing off the information below and giving it to a friend.

Dennis Richard has posted videos that will help you better understand some of the things discussed in *Your Health Is Your Choice*. To view them, go to:

www.YourHealthisYourChoice.org / www.DrHealth.com / www.DRhealthclub.com

Or go to **www.youtube.com and search for DennisRichard-books and MMSdr1**

Please help me with the distribution of my book by tearing off the information below and giving it to a friend.

Dennis Richard has posted videos that will help you better understand some of the things discussed in *Your Health Is Your Choice*. To view them, go to:

www.YourHealthisYourChoice.org / www.DrHealth.com / www.DRhealthclub.com

Or go to **www.youtube.com and search for DennisRichard-books and MMSdr1**

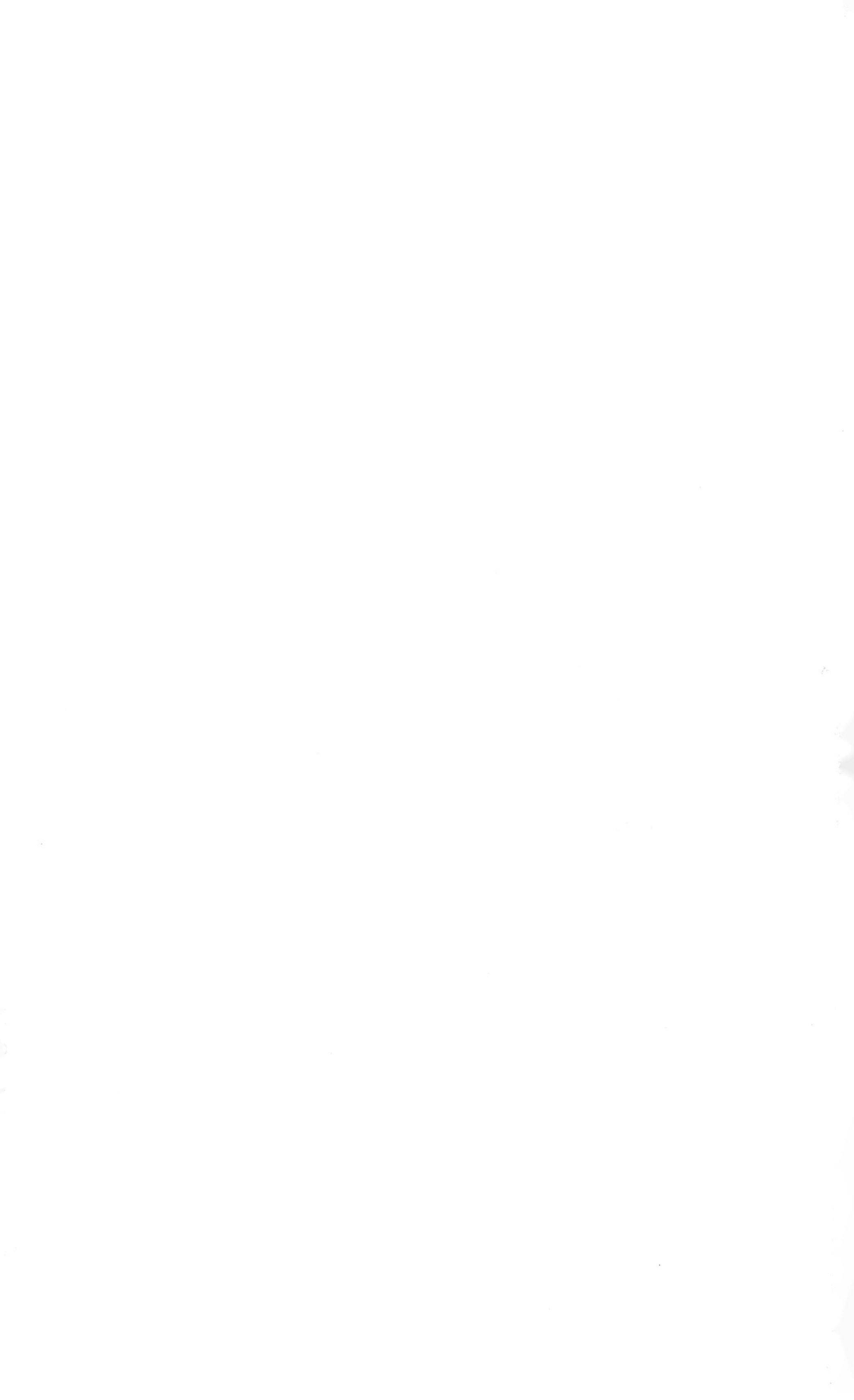

Made in the USA
San Bernardino, CA
06 May 2015